EAT, LEARN, REMEMBER

Edited by **Aise Seda Artis**

Eat, Learn, Remember
http://dx.doi.org/10.5772/intechopen.73147
Edited by Aise Seda Artis

Contributors

Genaro Gabriel Ortiz, Oscar Kurt Bitzer-Quintero, Luis Humberto De Loera-Rodríguez, Daniela Lucero Del Carmen Delgado-Lara, Jose A Cruz-Serrano, Erandis D Tórres-Sánchez, Miriam A Mora-Navarro, I. Gabriela Ortiz-Velázquez, Héctor González-Usigli, Mario Mireles-Ramírez, Michele Tine, Sophie Lenihan, Clara Batchelder, Regina Guarnieri, Orlando Bueno, Ivanda Tudesco, Aise Seda Artis

First published in London, United Kingdom, 2019 by IntechOpen
IntechOpen is the global imprint of INTECHOPEN LIMITED, registered in England and Wales, registration number: 11086078, The Shard, 25th floor, 32 London Bridge Street
London, SE19SG – United Kingdom
Printed in Croatia

British Library Cataloguing-in-Publication Data
A catalogue record for this book is available from the British Library

Additional hard copies can be obtained from orders@intechopen.com

Eat, Learn, Remember, Edited by Aise Seda Artis
p. cm.
Print ISBN 978-1-78985-165-6
Online ISBN 978-1-78985-166-3

For EU product safety concerns:
IN TECH d.o.o., Prolaz Marije Krucifikse Kozulić 3, 51000 Rijeka, Croatia,
info@intechopen.com or visit our website at intechopen.com.

Meet the editor

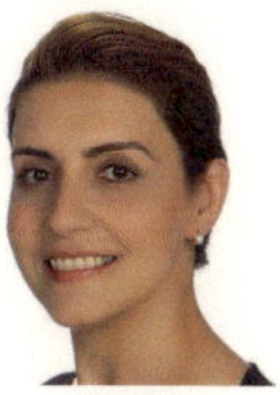

Aise Seda Artis, MD, is an Associate Professor of Physiology. She graduated from Istanbul University Cerrahpasa School of Medicine, Istanbul, Turkey, in 1998. She had experience at different clinics in Turkey and the USA as a general practitioner or researcher. During her training in Physiology at Erciyes University School of Medicine, Kayseri, Turkey, she had the opportunity to be involved in neuroscience. After training, she worked at the same department as an academic staff member. She then continued her academic career at Istanbul Medeniyet University School of Medicine, Istanbul, Turkey. At present she is working as a medical director of a pharmaceutical company.

Contents

Preface

Memory is a constructive process through which we actively organize and shape information. We say that it resembles computers, but living memory is flexible and capable of constant change. Encoding, storage, and retrieval processes are still not defined and understood clearly. Human memories are often fuzzy and fragile.

For years, learning and memory in animal models have been widely assessed in scientific research, trying to figure out their mechanisms. There is a diversity of experimental methods assessing animal learning and memory skills from the molecular level to mazes. Besides different in vivo and in vitro techniques, organ-on-a-chip technology is now also available. Various methods also have been developed to evaluate memory in humans, such as magnetic resonance imaging, memory tasks, and electrophysiological and neurophysiological tests. Also, computer-based technologies such as use of virtual reality provide an advantage. All those scientific efforts are spent for the sake of improving the way we learn and remember.

This book aims to reflect a taste of the accumulated knowledge.

I would like to thank Author Service Manager Ms. Romina Rovan and Commissioning Editor Ms. Lucija Tomicic-Dromgool for their constant help, patience, and kindness. Lastly, I shouldn't forget to mention Author Service Manager Ms. Martina Brkljacic who joined the team towards the end of the project. Those hardworking ladies prioritizing science before most other things made me feel a member of the growing IntechOpen family.

Aise Seda Artis, MD
Associate Professor of Medical Physiology
Istanbul Medeniyet University, Istanbul, Turkey

Chapter 1

Introductory Chapter: Eat, Learn, Remember

Aise Seda Artis

Additional information is available at the end of the chapter

http://dx.doi.org/10.5772/intechopen.82365

"Cogito ergo sum"

"I think, therefore I am"

René Descartes

1. Introduction

Is act of thinking simply enough to prove existence? At the age of artificial intelligence (AI) and virtual (VR) while talking about machine learning (ML), deep learning (DL), and Internet of Things (IoT), it is not easy to answer that.

What should be the proof that it is not a robot but a human being? Can it be the consciousness, being conscious of self-thoughts? According to Amit Goswami, consciousness is the ground of being. It is the continuing stream of awareness of surroundings or sequential thoughts, the highest state of awareness anyone can attain. It helps us learn and adapt to changing circumstances far more rapidly and effectively. On the other hand, the key to consciousness is the memory. Newly discovered neuronal rosehip cells might be the exact answer to the question by time [1]. Rosehip cells might be helping us to form memories, the building blocks of our existence.

2. Memory hypothesis

Maybe the best definition of memory is done by Oscar Wilde: "Memory is the diary that we all carry with us." It is simple, yet comprehensive. Memory is mainly the outcome of learning. Here, learning refers to the process by which experiences change our nervous system and hence our behavior.

Today, what we know at present is just a small piece of the phenomenal mechanism of memory. Every person's brain holds billions of bits of information. In order to remember, the information needs to be encoded, stored, and retrieved. Long-term memory has a vast, difficult-to-estimate capacity. We routinely access this data store shorter than the blink of an eye. Actually, memory is both a result of and an influence on perception, attention, and learning. We can hold onto some memories for hours or days, even without constant rehearsal—such as the scheduled time of a luncheon or the place we parked our car before leaving for a vacation. Furthermore, the time needed for consolidation varies enormously depending on our interest and/or previous familiarity with the topic.

The other edge of the sword is forgetting. Forgetfulness is sometimes a blessing physiological event, and sometimes part of a serious pathology, e.g., Alzheimer's disease (AD). The most common causes of memory loss are dementia, depression, stress, sleep deprivation, nutritional deficiency, medications, alcohol, tobacco, drug use, head injury, and stroke. Amnesia, a partial or total loss of memory, can be either of two types: One is retrograde amnesia, meaning amnesia for events that preceded some disturbance to the brain, such as a head injury or electroconvulsive shock. Damage in the thalamic areas may cause retrograde amnesia. The other type is anterograde amnesia, referring to amnesia for events that occur after some disturbance to the brain, such as head injury or certain degenerative brain diseases. Hippocampal lesions may also be the reason. Hippocampi are important in learning, but not for reflexive (skill) learning. Hippocampus and medial thalamic nuclei play a role in limbic thoughts (reward and punishment). People with anterograde amnesia are unable to consolidate information about location of rooms, corridors, buildings, roads, and other important items in their environment. The ability to remember the position or location of objects and places is called the spatial memory. Spatial memory has representations within working, short-term and long-term memory. It is sometimes considered in the context of episodic memory, one type of declarative memory. Bilateral medial temporal lobe lesions produce most profound impairment in spatial memory, but significant deficits can be produced by damage that is limited to the right hemisphere [2].

Long-term memory is often divided into two further main types: explicit (or declarative) memory and implicit (or procedural, nondeclarative) memory. By definition declarative memory is the memory that can be verbally expressed, such as memory for events in a person's past ("knowing what"). On the other hand, nondeclarative memory is a collective term for perceptual, stimulus-response, and motor memory ("knowing how"). In that case, the memory formation does not depend on hippocampal formation, located in the temporal lobe of each cerebral cortex. The term hippocampal formation typically refers to the dentate gyrus, the hippocampus proper (i.e., cornu ammonis), and the subicular cortex.

Information transfer within the nervous system is basically provided by the nerve cells. Neurons are the basic units of the nervous system. The synapse, the connection of two neurons, is the functional unit of the brain. Physiologically, memories are stored in the brain by changing the basic sensitivity of synaptic transmission between neurons as a result of the previous neural activity. New or facilitated synaptic pathways are called memory traces that can occur at all levels of the brain. A memory trace, also known as an engram, is a theoretical means by which memories are physically stored in the brain. All memories are not processed through the same steps. There are different neural mechanisms mediating several types of memory, all of which is caused by electrochemical and structural changes within the synapses. Common to all forms of memory is the cellular and circuitry changes in the nervous system. To understand the mechanisms underlying learning and memory that involve changes at the molecular, cellular, and network levels is still a major goal for neuroscientists.

Learning does not occur through a single way; it can take at least four basic forms:

1. Perceptual learning: Learning to recognize a particular stimulus. Perceptual learning involves learning to recognize things, not what to do when they are present. It can involve learning to recognize entirely new stimuli, or it can involve learning to recognize changes or variations in familiar stimuli.
2. Stimulus-response learning: Learning to automatically make a particular response in the presence of particular stimulus includes classical and instrumental conditioning.
3. Motor learning: Learning to make a new response
4. Relational learning: Learning relationships among individual stimuli. It is commonly classified into:
   a. Spatial learning
   b. Episodic learning
   c. Observational learning

Learning and memory are strongly associated with electrical activity in neurons, particularly in the hippocampus. We can study learning and memory in hippocampal neurons by examining how they respond to different patterns of input. To investigate brain mechanisms involved in identifying the origin of memories, event-related potentials (ERPs), long-term potentiation (LTP), and long-term depression (LTD) are recorded. While ERPs are used for humans, LTP and LTD are appropriate and commonly used to describe changes in cellular mechanisms underlying synaptic plasticity mainly used for synaptic plasticity at in vitro and in vivo rodent studies [3].

The synaptic plasticity and memory hypothesis have been a subject of interest for many scientists. The idea that learning results from changes in the strength of the synapse was first suggested by Cajal at the end of the nineteenth century based on insights from his anatomical studies. Hebb developed more refined models in the 1940s and defined the modulation of synaptic connectivity as a critical mechanism of learning. For the experimental purposes, in order to examine changes in the neuronal components of a specific behavior during or after the modification of that behavior with learning, different behavioral systems were developed [4]. The first models helped to define the neuronal changes that underlie learning and memory through simple forms of procedural memory such as habituation, sensitization, and classical conditioning. *Aplysia* gill-withdrawal reflex is maybe the best known among these models emerged at 1963 by Kandel and Tauc. By allowing electrophysiological recording from individual neurons, these systems provided the first experimental insight into the cellular mechanisms of memory [4, 5].

Modulation of neurotransmitter release changes synaptic strength, and this is a mechanism learning and short-term memory. It is well demonstrated in both the gill-withdrawal reflex of *Aplysia* and in the tail-flick response of crayfish. The plasticity occurred at the sensory neuron inputs onto the motor neurons that control the reflex response and thus directly modulate its magnitude. The results showed that clear structural changes in both the pre- and postsynaptic cells can accompany even elementary forms of learning and memory. Memory storage does not depend on specialized, superimposed memory neurons whose only function is to store rather than process information. The sensory-to-motor neuron synapses playing a role in the gill-withdrawal reflex are also the cellular substrates of learning and memory. The capability of memory storage is built into the neural architecture of the reflex pathway [4].

Stimulation with a high-frequency train of action potentials was shown to produce a prolonged strengthening of synaptic transmission that is called long-term potentiation (LTP), in all three of the major hippocampal pathways [4]. N-Methyl-D-aspartate (NMDA) and alpha-amino-3-hydroxy-5-methyl-4-isoxazole propionic acid (AMPA)-type glutamate receptors (NMDARs, AMPARs) are ionotropic receptors and important for synaptic plasticity [6]. NMDA receptors control Ca^{2+} channel that is normally blocked by Mg^{2+} ions. They are blocked by a drug called AP5 (2-amino-5-phosphonopentanoate). AMPA receptors control Na^{+} channel. The early phases of expression are mediated by a redistribution of AMPARs. When open, they produce excitatory postsynaptic potentials (EPSPs). Evoked potential that represents EPSPs of population of neurons is called population EPSP [3].

LTP and long-term depression (LTD) are two forms of activity-dependent changes, and both are believed to represent cellular correlates of learning and memory [6]. LTP and LTD are induced by specific patterns of activity. Because NMDAR-dependent calcium influx induces both LTP and LTD, the cell must have a way to decide whether to potentiate or depress a synaptic connection. For LTP induction both pre- and postsynaptic neurons need to be active at the same time because the postsynaptic neuron must be depolarized when glutamate is released from the presynaptic bouton to fully relieve the Mg^{2+} block of NMDARs. Conversely, LTD can be induced by repeated activation of the presynaptic neuron at low frequencies without postsynaptic activity. LTP initiates as a predominant amplification of AMPARs [7]. But the behavior of NMDA can largely explain the critical features of LTP: synapse specificity, cooperativity, and associativity. Unlike most neurotransmitter receptors that respond simply to the presence or absence of their cognate transmitter in the synaptic cleft, the NMDA receptor is also sensitive to the state of the postsynaptic membrane in which it resides.

Besides electrophysiology, electrochemical methods like voltammetry are versatile tools for detecting, monitoring, and measuring various neurochemical species. The "gold standard" for assessing ion-channel function is the patch-clamp electrophysiological technique on millisecond timescales with up to single channel resolution. Histopathological tests including immunohistochemistry and immunofluorescence give important clues to neuroscientists [8–10]. Cognitive behavioral and neuroimaging (among them most useful being functional magnetic resonance imaging (fMRI)) techniques are also commonly used [11]. Common behavioral testing paradigms for animal memory are fear conditioning, passive avoidance, object recognition, place learning and cue discrimination, water maze, and other mazes like T-maze and radial arm mazes [12]. Cognitive neuroscience aims to reduce cognition to its neural basis using newer technologies such as fMRI, repetitive transcranial magnetic stimulation (rTMS), and magnetoencephalography (MEG) as well as older methods such as positron emission tomography (PET) and electroencephalography (EEG) studies [13].

Although it is now clear that long-term synaptic plasticity is a key step in memory storage, it is important to note that to store a complex memory, changes in synaptic function must occur within the context of an ensemble of neurons to produce a specific alteration in information flow through a neural circuit. A second important challenge is to understand how the basic processes of memory storage are altered with age or disease, including AD. It becomes of critical importance to understand in sufficient detail both the basic mechanisms of memory storage and the changes that take place in disease to design specific compounds that can be used to restore cognitive function [4].

3. Eat

In the early 1800s, continental Europeans like Savarin verbalized the idea of "you are what you eat" that has been preached at the East for centuries. The mucosa of the gastrointestinal tract is the largest surface that interacts with the external environment. The gastrointestinal tract contains approximately 500 million neurons which collectively constitute the enteric nervous system and represent in total numbers as much as that contained in the spinal cord. Intrinsic primary afferent neurons (IPANs) that form 20% of the enteric neurons comprise in the detection of certain inflammatory mediators and inflammation with the gastrointestinal tract [14].

Inhibiting nitric oxide (NO) synthesis during learning that food is inedible in *Aplysia* blocks subsequent memory formation. Memory that food is inedible arises in three steps: (1) chemoreceptors responding to food on the lips, (2) receptors signaling active efforts to swallow food within the mouth, and (3) receptors signaling differential gut responses to success or failure to swallow [15].

On the other hand, a growing body of preclinical literature has demonstrated bidirectional signaling between the brain and the gut microbiome, involving multiple neurocrine and endocrine signaling mechanisms [16]. Li et al. observed a correlation between dietary-induced shifts in bacteria diversity and animal behavior that may indicate a role for gut bacterial diversity in memory and learning [14]. Studies have shown that protein-induced proliferation of gut bacteria in mice augments spatial memory, and the ingestion of probiotic mixtures by healthy volunteers improves problem-solving abilities and has anxiolytic actions [17, 18]. Recent findings have resulted in speculation that alterations in the gut microbiome may play a pathophysiological role in human brain diseases, including autism spectrum disorder, anxiety, depression, chronic pain, obsessive-compulsive disorder, and memory abilities (including spatial and nonspatial memory) [16, 19].

4. Learn

It is well established that the hippocampus is one of the most important brain structures involved in learning; and lesions in this area cause impairment in learning, with location and severity of lesion influencing the severity of the effect on learning. But it has been proven that even in the absence of the hippocampus, learning can still occur. This suggests that other brain areas like the amygdala and olfactory bulb also play a role in the formation of new memories [12].

It is an important challenge to understand how the basic processes of memory storage are altered with age or disease, such as AD. It becomes of critical importance to understand in sufficient detail both the basic mechanisms of memory storage and the changes that take place in disease to design specific compounds that can be used to restore cognitive function [4]. The presence of amyloid plaques and neurofibrillary tangles in histological sections of the brain is required for the definitive diagnosis of AD. The cognitive decline is observed earlier than the visualization of the plaques. Amyloid-β peptide (Aβ) is the major component of the amyloid plaques. A large body of evidence accumulated in the past 15 years supports a pivotal role of soluble Aβ oligomers (AβOs) in synapse failure and neuronal dysfunction, disrupting LTP and LTD mechanisms in AD [6, 20].

Through varied mechanisms, gut microbes shape the architecture of sleep and stress reactivity of the hypothalamic-pituitary-adrenal axis. They influence memory, mood, and cognition and are clinically and therapeutically relevant to a range of disorders, including celiac disease, alcoholism, chronic fatigue syndrome, fibromyalgia, restless legs syndrome, and multiple sclerosis (MS) [21]. MS involves an immune-mediated process in which an abnormal response of the body's immune system is directed against the central nervous system, causing chronic inflammatory demyelinating disease. Since gut microorganisms play an important role in the development of the autoimmune system and are associated with a variety of autoimmune and metabolic diseases, it is speculated that gut symbiotic microorganisms play an important role in the susceptibility to MS [22].

Parkinson's disease (PD) follows a defined clinical pattern, and a range of nonmotor symptoms precede the motor phase. Evidence suggests that environmental factors have an important role in triggering and/or propagating the pathology of PD; the olfactory and gastrointestinal systems are gateways to the environment. The neurodegeneration process that leads to PD seems to start in the ENS or the olfactory bulb. The intricate relationship of governing host and microorganism interactions suggests that when this relationship is abnormal, the microorganisms may cause the pathogenesis of disease or promote the progression of disease. The microbiota may alter adult hippocampal neurogenesis. Hippocampus and lateral ventricle have the function of generating new neurons in adulthood. Adult hippocampal neurogenesis has a role in learning and memory and can affect the pathogenesis of many neurological disorder-related diseases and symptoms, such as epilepsy, depression, AD, and Parkinson's disease (PD) [23].

http://dx.doi.org/10.5772/intechopen.82365

5. Remember

"Remembering the past is a form of mental time travel: it frees us from the constraints of time and space and allows us to move freely along completely different dimensions" said Eric Kandel. Learning is a behavioral change due to an experience. Memory is storage and recall of information. It is widely accepted that learning process consists of at least two stages: short-term memory and long-term memory. Models of memory include distinctions among very short-lived memories like sensory memory, which has a lifetime measured in milliseconds to seconds; short- to medium-lived memories like short-term memory and working memory, which persist for seconds to minutes; and memories that may persist for decades, which we call long-term memory. Working memory is often referred to as a mental juggler, because it is what allows the brain to do many different things at once. And, memory itself can be broken down into two types: explicit and implicit. Explicit (or declarative) memory is recall of personal events/personal facts (episodic memory) or recall of facts (semantic memory). Implicit (or nondeclarative) memory is recall of reflexive motor skills or perceptual skills.

The rule of thumb for memory is "use it or lose it." Forgetting might be a problem; but sometimes the thing we remember might cause the trouble. One of the major problems in memory research in humans is its fallible nature. Having the ability to recall memories does not necessarily mean they are accurate. Our ability to store and process what is going on and using the classified information basically relies on memory being a constructive, fallible process. Children's memory is more susceptible to suggesting and implanting of false memories than adults. Since the underlying neurophysiological mechanisms for such an association are similar to the one that occurs when a genuine memory is formed, it is not surprising that the subject behaves as if the (false) memory was formed by a perceived real experience [24]. The formation of false memories in humans often occurs as a result of recombining mnemonic elements of discrete experiences into a new, reconstructed memory that is not a veridical representation of the past. These memories are not formed de novo and require pre-existing memories as a platform onto which distinct experiences can be incorporated to update the memory itself [24].

6. Conclusion

Recently, memory research has accelerated and we have seen an explosion of new knowledge in neuroscience. A set of persuasive evidence for the long-sought memory engram and engram cells has now come of age. The evidence has been obtained by combining multiple technologies, each addressing a specific level of complexity. Here, you will read a tiny part of the accumulated knowledge to elucidate the usefulness and limitations of these into clinical practice and daily life.

Eat to live, live to learn, and remember to value everything just as much as they deserve.

Acknowledgements

I would like to thank Author Service Manager Ms. Romina Rovan and Commissioning Editor Ms. Lucija Tomicic-Dromgool for their constant help and patience.

Author details

Aise Seda Artis

Address all correspondence to: aseda@yahoo.com

Istanbul Medeniyet University, Istanbul, Turkey

References

[1] Boldog E, Bakken T, Hodge RD, Novotny M, Aevermann BD, Baka J, et al. Transcriptomic and morphophysiological evidence for a specialized human cortical GABAergic cell type. Nature Neuroscience. 2018 Sep;**21**(9):1185-1195

[2] Buffalo EA, Bellgowan PSF, Martin A. Distinct roles for medial temporal lobe structures in memory for objects and their locations. Learning & Memory; 2006;**13**(5):638-643

[3] Purves D, Augustine GJ, Fitzpatrick D, Katz LC, LaMantia A-S, McNamara JO, et al. Neuroscience. 3rd ed. Sunderland, MA, USA: Sinauer Associates, Inc.; 2004

[4] Mayford M, Siegelbaum SA, Kandel ER. Synapses and memory storage. Cold Spring Harbor Perspectives in Biology; 2012 Jun 1;**4**(6). pii: a005751

[5] Lisman J, Cooper K, Sehgal M, Silva AJ. Memory formation depends on both synapse-specific modifications of synaptic strength and cell-specific increases in excitability. Nature Neuroscience; 2018 Mar;**21**(3):309-314

[6] Lüscher C, Malenka RC. NMDA receptor-dependent long-term potentiation and long-term depression (LTP/LTD). Cold Spring Harbor Perspectives in Biology; 2012;**4**(6): a005710

[7] Dozmorov M, Li R, Abbas AK, Hellberg F, Farre C, Huang FS, et al. Contribution of AMPA and NMDA receptors to early and late phases of LTP in hippocampal slices. Neuroscience Research; 2006 Jun;**55**(2):182-188

[8] Borland LM, Michael AC. An introduction to electrochemical methods in neuroscience. Michael AC, Borland LM, Editors. In: Electrochemical Methods for Neuroscience. Florida, USA: CRC Press; 2007

[9] Accardi MV, Pugsley MK, Forster R, Troncy E, Huang H, Authier S. The emerging role of in vitro electrophysiological methods in CNS safety pharmacology. Journal of Pharmacological and Toxicological Methods; 2016 Sep-Oct;**81**:47-59

[10] Lin AL, Monica Way HY. Functional magnetic resonance imaging. McManus LM, Mitchell RN, editors. In: Pathobiology of Human Disease. MA, USA: Academic Press, Elsevier Inc.; 2014

[11] Weingarten CP, Strauman TJ. Neuroimaging for psychotherapy research: Current trends. Psychotherapy Research; 2015;**25**(2):185-213

[12] Savage S, Ma D. Animal behaviour testing: Memory. British Journal of Anaesthesia; 2014 Jul;**113**(1):6-9

[13] Kable JW. The cognitive neuroscience toolkit for the neuroeconomist: A functional overview. Journal of Neuroscience, Psychology, and Economics; 2011;**4**(2):63-84

[14] Li W, Dowd SE, Scurlock B, Acosta-Martinez V, Lyte M. Memory and learning behavior in mice is temporally associated with diet-induced alterations in gut bacteria. Physiology & Behavior; 2009 Mar 23;**96**(4-5):557-567

[15] Katzoff A, Miller N, Susswein AJ. Nitric oxide and histamine signal attempts to swallow: A component of learning that food is inedible in Aplysia. Learn Memory. 2009 Dec 30;**17**(1):50-62

[16] Mayer EA, Knight R, Mazmanian SK, Cryan JF, Tillisch K. Gut microbes and the brain: Paradigm shift in neuroscience. The Journal of Neuroscience; 2014 Nov 12;**34**(46):15490-15496

[17] Bravo JA, Forsythe P, Chew MV, Escaravage E, Savignac HM, Dinan TG, et al. Ingestion of Lactobacillus strain regulates emotional behavior and central GABA receptor expression in a mouse via the vagus nerve. USA: Proceedings of the National Academy of Sciences; 2011 Sep 20;**108**(38):16050-16055

[18] Burnet PWJ. Gut bacteria and brain function: The challenges of a growing field. USA: Proceedings of the National Academy of Sciences; 2012 Jan 24;**109**(4):E176

[19] Wang H, Lee IS, Braun C, Enck P. Effect of probiotics on central nervous system functions in animals and humans: A systematic review. Journal of Neurogastroenterology and Motility; 2016 Oct 30;**22**(4):589-605

[20] Ferreira ST, Lourenco MV, Oliveira MM, De Felice FG. Soluble amyloid-β oligomers as synaptotoxins leading to cognitive impairment in Alzheimer's disease. Frontiers in Cellular Neuroscience; 2015 May 26;**9**:191

[21] Galland L. The gut microbiome and the brain. Journal of Medicinal Food; 2014 Dec;**17**(12):1261-1272

[22] Zhu X, Han Y, Du J, Liu R, Jin K, Yi W. Microbiota-gut-brain axis and the central nervous system. Oncotarget; 2017 May 10;**8**(32):53829-53838

[23] Mu Y, Gage FH. Adult hippocampal neurogenesis and its role in Alzheimer's disease. Molecular Neurodegeneration; 2011 Dec 22;**6**:85

[24] Tonegawa S, Liu X, Ramirez S, Redondo R. Memory engram cells have come of age. Neuron; 2015 Sep 2;**87**(5):918-931

Chapter 2

Gut-Brain Axis: Role of Microbiota in Parkinson's Disease and Multiple Sclerosis

Genaro Gabriel Ortiz, Loera-Rodriguez Luis H. de,
José A. Cruz-Serrano, Erandis D. Torres-Sánchez,
Miriam A. Mora-Navarro,
Daniela L. C. Delgado-Lara,
Irma Gabriela Ortiz-Velázquez,
Héctor González-Usigli,
Oscar K. Bitzer-Quintero and Mario Mireles Ramírez

Additional information is available at the end of the chapter

http://dx.doi.org/10.5772/intechopen.79493

Abstract

It has recently been discovered that the digestive tract is lined with about 100 million nerve cells; the digestive tract has been baptized, metaphorically speaking, as "the second brain," which contains a multitude of neurotransmitters, viruses, and bacteria that help regulate our emotional state. This second brain, known as the enteric nervous system, is a unique anatomical unit that extends from the esophagus to the anus. Like the nervous system, it produces a whole series of psychoactive substances, such as serotonin, dopamine, and opioids for pain, and synthesizes benzodiazepines. In it, we find the microbiota: a set of microorganisms (viruses and bacteria). Together with the brain, the microbiota directly influences mood, character, or sleep. Knowledge about the possible relationship of the microbiota with frequent neurological diseases is still just beginning. Recently, possible changes in the microbiota have been linked to the onset of Parkinson's disease (PD). Also, today, we know that there are differences between the microbiota of healthy people and people with multiple sclerosis and that these differences have also been related to the disease and its evolution.

Keywords: brain, intestine, microbiota, neurodegeneration

1. Introduction

Currently, we know that the enteric nervous system, although it has a certain sovereignty or autonomy, will always need to communicate with other systems in order to carry out functions of its authorship or of other adjacent systems. Thus, in a classical way, the enteric nervous system interacts with the central nervous system but also exhibits a certain exchange of stimuli with other systems. Through this connection afferent and efferent responses are generated, with the consequent exchange of information. Remember that the afferent neurons send information of the intraluminal chemical content, mechanical state of the intestinal wall, and tissue situation (inflammation, pH, cold, and heat) to the central nervous system. The responses follow an extrinsic efferent pathway where the main neurotransmitter is norepinephrine. In addition, the efferent neurons come from the prevertebral nodes that control motility and secretion and the paravertebrals that control the flow of gastrointestinal blood vessels. Also, the relaxation of the gastric *fundus* and gastric and pancreatic secretion is mediated through vagal neurons. In contrast to what happens in the upper digestive tract, the distal colon and rectum are innervated by pelvic nerves. In general, vagal stimulation inhibits motor activity, gastrointestinal secretion, sphincter contraction, and blood flow, while, on the contrary, spinal stimulation stimulates them. The responses may have extrinsic afferent pathways where spinal and vagal reflexes are also activated. The primary afferent vagal neurons have their cell bodies in the nodosum and jugular ganglia and project medially to the brain, while the spinal neuronal bodies are found in the roots of the dorsal ganglia. The vagal pathways transmit information about the physiological state of the digestive organs and regulate inflammatory responses, while the spinal pathways transmit the painful impulses.

2. Gut microbiota

Since 2007, the genome of 500 bacterial species that normally reside in the human intestine, and which together are known as microbiome or microbiota, has been identified. Our intestinal tract contains over 100 billion microbes, the vast majority in the colon, exceeding the number of human cells by a factor [1]. This complex microbial community is known as the gastrointestinal microbiota, and it consists of bacteria, *archaea*, eukaryotes, fungi, and viruses. Therefore, it has been proposed that the human being is a "meta-organism" with 10–100 times more bacterial than human cells, which integrate metabolically and immunologically. The composition of the microbiota, in addition to location, is influenced by age, sex, race, and other factors like diet, medication (especially antibiotics), stress, smoking, or gastrointestinal infections, as well as from each individual [2]. Even within each person, there are great variations in their composition if measured at different times. Although it is impossible to define the concept of healthy microbiota today, we do know that the richness and diversity of the microbiota are indicators of its health and that its impoverishment is associated with obesity and metabolic markers [2]. As for the qualitative composition, numerous studies are emerging that try to relate certain classes of microorganisms with different physiological states. It is proposed that there are those that improve the metabolic state, resistance to infections, cancer, autoimmunity, inflammation, endocrine signaling, and brain functionality

http://dx.doi.org/10.5772/intechopen.79493

(gut-brain axis): *Bacteroides, Bifidobacterium, Clostridium* group XIVa and IVa (butyrate producing), *Eubacterium, Faecalibacterium, Lactobacillus, and Roseburia* are considered today [3]. The relationship between the microbiota and the human being has been redefined from commensal to a mutualist relationship, where the bacteria provide biological functions not coded genetically in our organism, which go from metabolic activity to immunological homeostasis, considering the microbiota as a fundamental, virtual organ in the pathophysiological and immunological responses. There are studies related to the role of the intestinal microbiota in human health, infections, and neurological diseases [4] (**Figure 1**).

It has rarely been thought that microorganisms and the brain interact except in instances where pathogens penetrate the blood-brain barrier, which is the cellular strength that protects the brain from infections and inflammation [5]. When they do, they can have strong effects. Bidirectional communication between the brain-nervous system and the microbiota is well known in specific cases. Pavlov's experiments showed how a sound processed by the brain can condition the physiology of the digestive system, stimulating, among other things, gastric secretion [6].

Clostridium botulinum can colonize the intestine and from there release its toxin that blocks the release of acetylcholine at the neuromuscular synapse. In the case of hepatic encephalopathy, brain dysfunction is a consequence of substances produced in the intestine, and its treatment includes the use of antibiotics and probiotics [7]. Certain autoimmune neurological diseases, such as Guillain-Barré syndrome, may have their origin in certain intestinal bacteria and *Campylobacter jejuni.* The virus that causes rabies generates aggression, agitation, and even a fear of water, but for decades the vast majority of the body's natural microbes had not

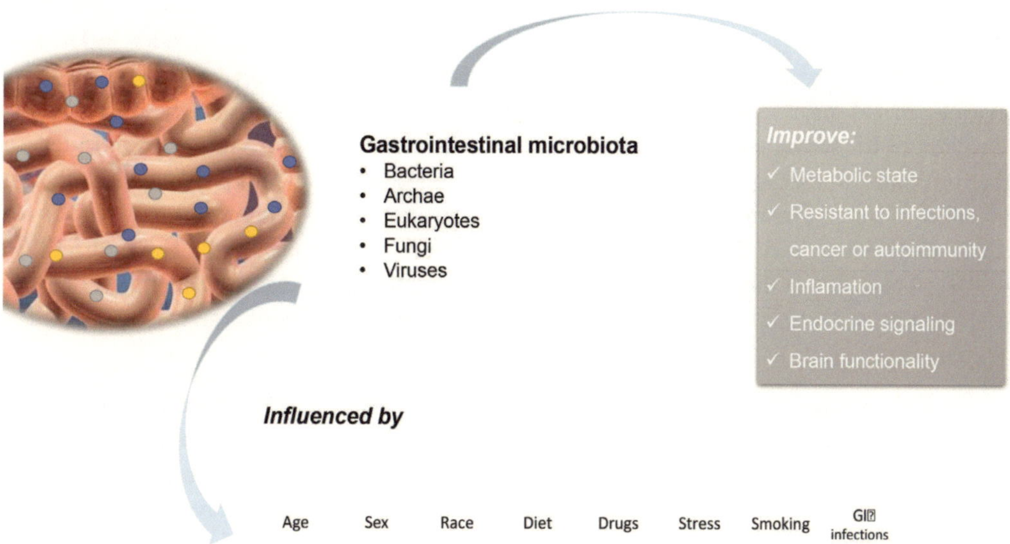

Figure 1. The composition of the intestinal microbiota is influenced by physicochemical conditions and also depends on the anatomical region along the GI. The type and number of microbial species that persist and colonize the GI tract are determined by a combination of factors including but not limited to the host genetics, medications, diet, environmental factors, and to the inflammatory state of the host. In elderly patients, we can observe changes in the composition of the microbiota in comparison to young people, which could lead to a dysbiosis.

been described, and while the idea that they could influence neurobiology hardly prevailed, that is slowly changing [8]. On the other hand, metabolic functions include the degradation of polysaccharides to short-chain fatty acids, such as butyrate, propionate, and acetate, with anti-inflammatory properties and the main energetic substrate of colonocytes, and thus are implicated in the barrier function of the gut mucosa [9]. Some bacteria, particularly *lactobacilli,* have been implicated in cholesterol metabolism and in the production of vitamins K and B and are also involved in the metabolism of xenobiotics, drugs, antibiotics, or bioactive products, conditioning pharmacokinetics, and the production of certain toxins involved in many diseases [9].

2.1. Microbiota and immune response

The microbiota contributes to various immunological functions. In the gut barrier, it prevents colonization and growth of pathogenic microorganisms, and it matures the immune barrier, both stimulating the innate response through Toll-like receptors (TLR) and NOD-like receptors (NLR) as the adaptive one, with an important role in the secretion of mucins, antimicrobial peptides, defensins, and IgA [10]. Regarding the development of the systemic immune response, in working with germ-free mice, the microbiota has been observed to intervene in the regulation and maturation of Peyer's plaques, mesenteric lymph nodes, and germinal centers [11]. It also regulates the number of plasma cells producing IgA, gut Tγδ cells, and CD4 + T lymphocytes in the lamina propria or intraepithelial and is involved in the gene expression of TLR and the major histocompatibility complex II [12]. The microbiota also conditions the development of effector T cells and the production of cytokines, highlighting the influence on Th and Treg lymphocytes involved in the autoimmune response and its regulation and, therefore, in autoimmune diseases in general and in multiple sclerosis in particular [13]. Germ-free mice (mice raised to lack intestinal microbiota) present a reduction in Th1 and Th lymphocytes, balancing the T-immune response to Th, which is reversed by reconstituting the normal gut microbiota in these animals. It has been proposed that the microbiota is involved in the passage of stationary T lymphocytes to pro-autoimmune T lymphocytes, so that mutualist microorganisms induce the production of Th at a steady state, which, in the presence of a proinflammatory microenvironment, promoted by certain cytokines such as IL-12, IL-23, IL-1β, or TGF-β3, would pass to pathogenic Th, a producer of IFN-γ, contributing to the progression of the inflammatory bowel environment [14]. It has been shown that the involvement of a single bacterium, the segmented filamentous bacteria, can contribute to this Th pro-autoimmune activity [14] (**Figure 2**).

As for the Treg, the microbiota is indispensable for its development and function. These lymphocytes regulate the inflammation that is generated against microbial stimuli through IL-10 [15]. Numerous microbial agents have been linked to the induction of Treg, notably the role of *Bacteroides fragilis* and specifically its polysaccharide A (PSA) with the development of IL-10 producing Foxp3+ regulatory T cells and with the prevention and cure of experimental colitis or shock in animal models, showing its key role in the regulation of immunological tolerance [16]. The aforementioned short-chain fatty acids, especially butyrate, balance the immune system to an "anti-inflammatory state" by increasing the production of IL-10 and IL-4, reducing

http://dx.doi.org/10.5772/intechopen.79493

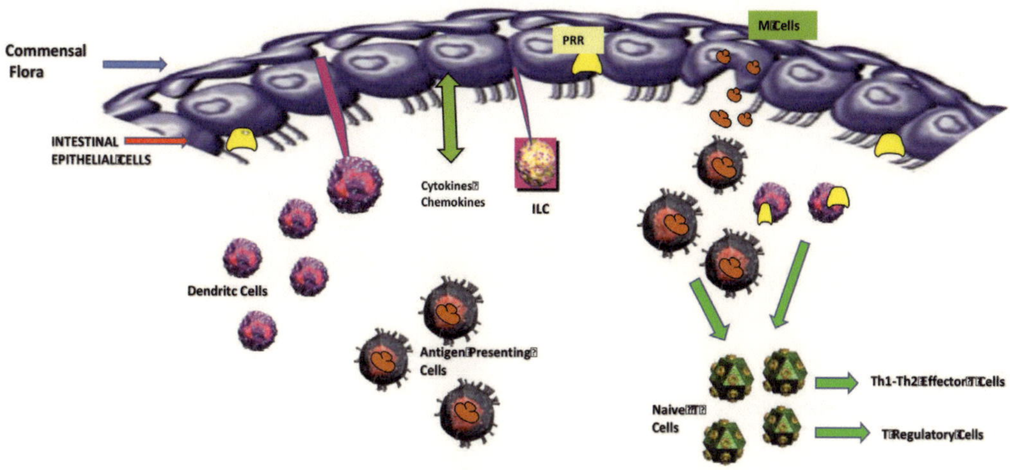

Figure 2. Microbiota stimulation leads to B cell switch to lga, regulatory T-cell induction, and T-cell differentiation to Th17. This image is a modification of QIAGEN's original at www.qiagen.com/mx/shop/genes-and-pathways/pathway-details/?pwid=468.

vascular adhesion of VCAM-mediated leukocytes, inhibiting function of IFN-γ and therefore its proinflammatory capacity, and regulating the Treg lymphocytes and the inflammatory function of leukocytes [17] (**Figure 3**).

2.2. Gut and nervous system

The surface of the gut mucosa is the most extensive of the organism and also houses the largest number of lymphoid structures in the human body. The innervations of the digestive tract are very abundant and are structured in three levels of plexus: functions of the enteric autonomic nervous system include bowel motility, vaso-regulation and permeability control, and secretion of certain gastroenteropancreatic hormones [18]. In addition, similar to what occurs in the blood-brain barrier, there are numerous astrocyte terminations at the border of the intestinal barrier that represent a potential pathway for communication with the rest of the nervous system. In the intestine we have about 100 million neurons, which are more than the spinal cord contains [19]. This multitude of neurons in the enteric nervous system allows us to feel the inner world of our gut and its contents. Much of this neuronal arsenal is evidenced in the elaborate daily routine of digestion, through decomposing food and absorbing nutrients. Expelling waste requires chemical, mechanical, and rhythmic muscle contractions that move everything to the end. Therefore, equipped with its own reflexes and senses, it can control the behavior of the gut independently of the brain. This nervous system of the intestine is connected to the brain in a bidirectional way. On one hand, the bowel receives information from the brain, and on the other hand, the bowel sends messages to the brain [20]. This communication of the intestine with the brain occurs both through the nervous system and the bloodstream and is called the gut-brain axis. Typical examples of this bidirectional circuit would be the increase in intestinal peristalsis (colicky pain and diarrhea) when our brain perceives a

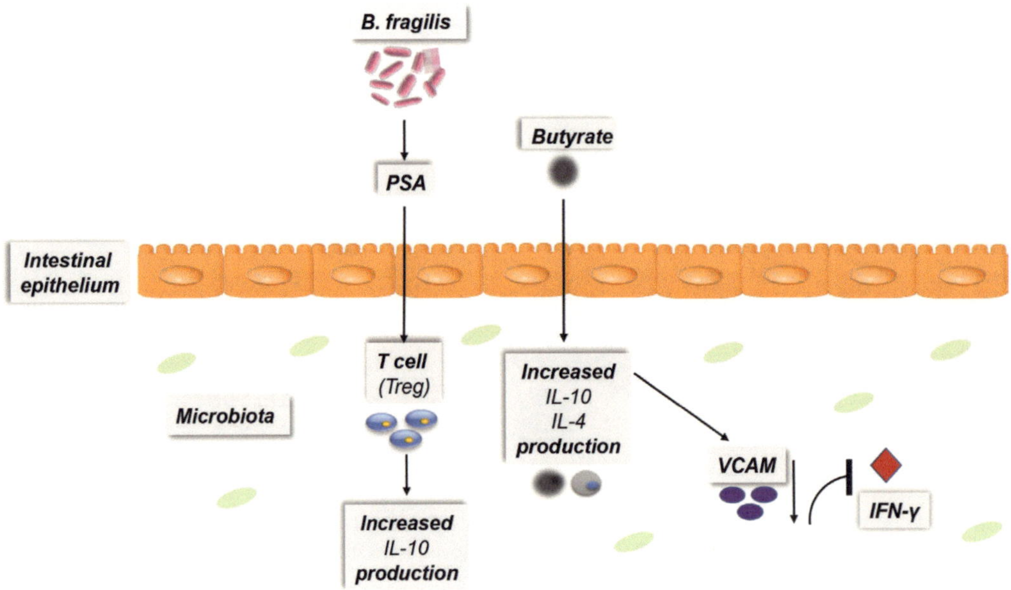

Figure 3. Regulation of inflammation by Treg, through IL-10 and IL-4 generated against microbial stimuli, *Bacteroides fragilis* specifically its polysaccharide a (PSA).

danger or, in the opposite direction, the sensation of satiety that our brain perceives when we have ingested a certain quantity of food [20] (**Figure 4**).

The intestine, besides having a nervous system of its own, is also an ecosystem. Colonization by the intestinal microbiota affects the brain development of mammals and their behavior during adulthood [21]. Through measurements of motor activity and behavior related to anxiety, it has been demonstrated in mice that the microbial colonization process triggers signaling mechanisms that affect these neural circuits, so that the gut microbiota can influence normal brain development and behavioral functions [22], and the microbiota is capable of modifying the expression of some risk genes or is part of the mechanisms that alter the cognitive functions observed in patients with gastrointestinal diseases [22]. The alteration of this microbiota and gut-brain axis could explain some of the mechanisms of the pathogenesis of diverse cerebral diseases like, for example, Parkinson's disease, multiple sclerosis, depression, Alzheimer's disease, etc., although today its etiology still remains unknown [23]. In studies in mice, it has been shown that alterations in the intestinal microbiota could be responsible for alterations in social behavior and that supplementation with probiotics such as *B. fragilis* administered in the early stages of adolescence in mice could reduce brain alterations [23]. But the influence of the microbiota on the brain is unknown in detail, beyond the simple examples previously uncovered, which do not reflect the full extent of this relationship. Much more articulate is the observation of what happens to mice whose digestive tract has remained sterile throughout their development as "germ-free" [23]. It has been found that in these animals the microglia does not mature properly and it is very difficult to provoke experimental allergic encephalitis and that these mice also have changes in their behavior, with increased responses to stress, and most amazingly, certain areas of their brain, like the amygdala and hippocampus, show structural differences.

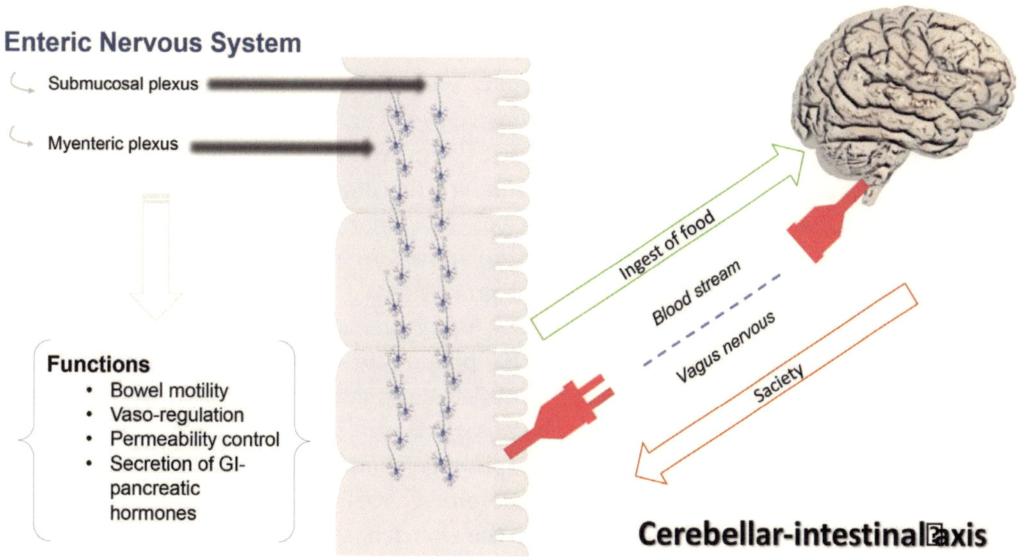

Figure 4. Key aspects of gastrointestinal physiology are controlled by the enteric nervous system, which is composed of neurons and glial cells. These cells of the enteric nervous system are connected to the central nervous system (in a bidirectional way). As an example, when we ingest food, through neural pathways and immune and endocrine mechanisms, we will perceive the sensation of satiety.

Given the role of the *vagus* nerve in the communication of signals between the gut and the brain, many investigations that seek to explore the connections between microorganisms and the CNS have examined the function of this nerve. Thus, it has been shown that both pathogenic and nonpathogenic bacteria appear to activate the *vagus* nerve. For example, subdiaphragmatic vagotomy attenuates the expression of c-fos in rats inoculated with *Salmonella typhimurium*; the combination of a *C. rodentium* infection and stress causes an increase in the activation of the vagal ganglion in mice; intraduodenal injection of *L. lactis* La1 activates the gastric vagal nerve in rats; subdiaphragmatic vagotomy blocks the anxiolytic and antidepressive effects of the chronic ingestion of *L. rhamnosus* in normal adult mice while avoiding the associated alterations in the expression of GABAAα2 mRNA in the amygdala; and vagotomy abolishes the ability of *B. longum* to attenuate anxiety induced by DSS colitis.

3. The second brain

The relationship between the brain, the emotions, and the digestive tract is intense. So much so that many scientists refer to the intestine as the "second brain" or "gut-brain," since the digestive tract contains a very complex neural network with a neuronal function very similar to the activity of the head.

The presence of receptors to various neurotransmitters in the intestine has been demonstrated: it is known that some intestinal molecules, such as serotonin 5-HT, can modulate the pathogenic potential of *Pseudomonas fluorescens* by affecting its motility and pyoverdine production but without affecting its growth. It has been reported that gut microbiota can control the tryptophan metabolism of the host by enhancing the fraction of tryptophan available for the kynurenine route and decreasing the amount available for 5-HT synthesis [24]. Free fatty acid receptor 3 (FFAR3) receptors for short-chain fatty acids (SCFAs) have been detected in submucosal and myenteric ganglia, and the responsiveness of enteric neurons to glucose, amino acids, and fatty acids has been demonstrated [24]. For example, there are receptors to the stress hormones epinephrine and norepinephrine, and this increases by more than four orders of magnitude in the human gut in the presence of *Clostridium/Bacteroides*. A recent report has demonstrated that *Vibrio cholerae* can respond to epinephrine and norepinephrine (enhancing the growth rate, swimming motility, and production of virulence factors such as iron sequestering phenotypes) by means of specific sensor proteins [24]. Less information is available on prokaryotic Glu receptors; however, 100 prokaryotic channel proteins with putative Glu-binding domains have recently been identified through a bioinformatic study. Among them, 22 proteins have been found to be homologs of vertebrate ionotropic Glu receptors. Multiple Glu receptor types (including ionotropic, types 1 and 4 metabotropic receptors, and heterodimeric TAS1R1 + TAS1R3, L-Glu taste receptors) have been detected in gastrointestinal (GI) epithelial cells and/or enteric neurons in the stomach, small intestine, and colon. And mGlu4 receptors have been detected in the mucosa of both the gastric *antrum* and duodenum, while both mGlu4 and mGlu7 receptors have been identified in the colon epithelium. A role of mGluRs in the human colon in the control of colon peristalsis and electrolyte transport has been described. High levels of mGlu7 and mGlu8 have been detected in myenteric neurons, where they are possibly involved in the regulation of gut motility [24]. The $GABA_B$ receptors are abundantly expressed in the GI tract. GABA and its ionotropic and metabotropic receptors are widely distributed throughout the ENS, in both submucosal and myenteric neurons, from the stomach to the ileum. The release of 5-HT by endothelial cells in the small intestine of guinea pig is modulated by $GABA_A$ and $GABA_B$ receptors. Involvement of $GABA_B$ receptors in modulation of sensitivity of vagal and spinal afferents has been reported [24].

To think that the intestine acts as a second brain is not something new if we look at the more oriental cultures [25]. For them, the belly was and is the center of the vital energy of the organism where they integrate mind and body. The small brain that we have in the gut works in connection with the big brain in the skull and partly determines our mental state and plays a key role in certain diseases that affect other parts of the body. In addition to neurons, all types of neurotransmitters in the brain are present in the digestive system. The enteric nervous system secretes the same substances as those found in our central nervous system. There are nerve pathways that specifically connect the brain areas related to our emotions and thoughts, the immune system, the endocrine system, and the enteric nervous system to each other. When there is a disfunction between any of these conected systems, pathological symptoms may appear in any of the others even without direct damage to them [25, 26] (**Figure 5**).

Is well known that 90% of total body serotonin is synthesized in the intestine and it has a direct implication in gastrointestinal physiology. In this sense, our diet is important because this serotonin is formed from a tryptophan, an essential amino acid, which is only obtained through food. Here we begin to see the relationship between the brain, the intestine, and the diet [27].

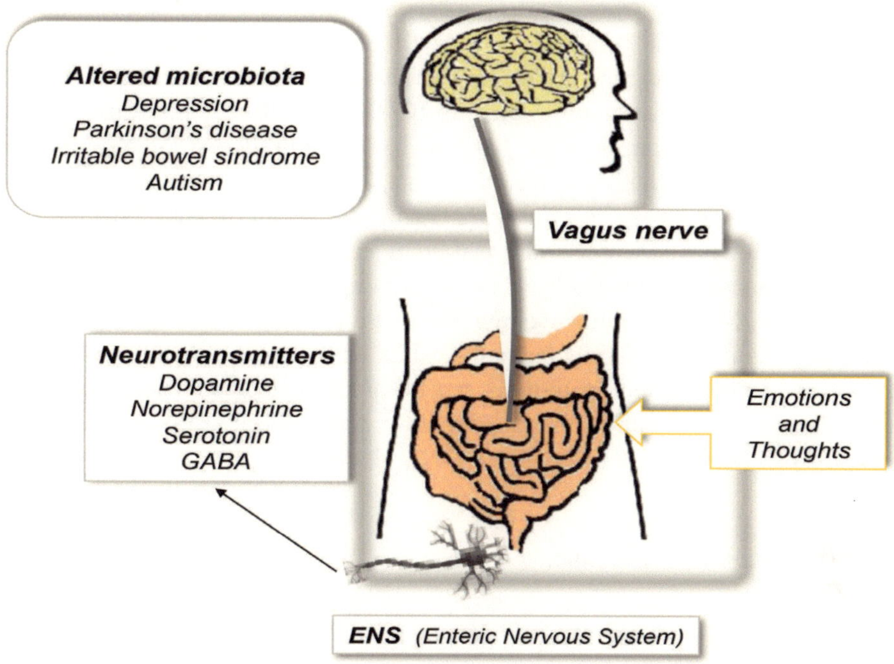

Figure 5. Second brain. In the intestine we can find neurotransmitters that are exported to the CNS.

3.1. Is the gut autonomous?

The gut has the ability to work in two ways: independently and in connection with the brain. This connection to the brain (gut-brain axis) is bidirectional in that it goes from the brain to the intestine and vice versa. We have long known that many emotional alterations, psychological issues, affect at the intestinal level, such as feelings, sadness, and loss of, or increase in, appetite. We mentioned above that serotonin in the intestine works as a neurotransmitter in the inhibition of anger, aggression, body temperature, mood, sleep, vomiting, and appetite and is responsible for keeping our state of equilibrium in balance (its different levels in our organism are related to depression). Here, more than 50% of the activity of dopamine also occurs: a neurotransmitter that among its functions regulates the levels of pleasure in our brain. Its secretion occurs during pleasant situations and encourages us to seek that activity or pleasing occupation. This means that food, sex, and various drugs are also stimulants for the secretion of dopamine in the brain in certain areas such as the nucleus accumbens and the prefrontal cortex [28].

3.2. Some other interactions in the gut-brain axis

Memory: the protein that burns the body fat is also responsible for memory, which is why obese people are more prone to dementia. **Well-being**: mood is lodged in the stomach since 90% of serotonin, the "happiness hormone," is produced and stored there. **Sleep**: when we relax the gut, our stomach neurons produce benzodiazepines that relax and induce sleep. **Stress:** in an emergency the brain takes energy from the bowel, and the guts send signals like upset stomach. **Gluttony:** the trillions of bacteria that lodge in the gut choose their own nutrients to thrive, and sometimes they are greedier than you. **Fear:** panic causes the brain to frighten the large intestine. It no longer has time to absorb fluid, and the result is diarrhea. The relationship between the brain, the microbiota, and the emotions is little investigated. There are very preliminary studies. Knowing exactly, at the clinical level, how it can impact is difficult to pin down. There are studies that point to the idea of using probiotics as a complementary treatment to drugs that treat anxiety or depressive disorders, as they may help amplify the effects, but this is still quite preliminary. Probiotics or foods rich in healthy bacteria, such as yogurts and other fermented milks, exhibited a positive influence on our behavior: *Lactobacillus* and *Bifidobacterium* bacteria are capable of producing gamma-aminobutyric acid, a neurotransmitter of the brain that regulates many psychological processes and whose dysfunction is related to anxiety and depression [29].

4. Neurodegenerative diseases

Knowledge of the possible relationship of the microbiota with frequent neurological diseases is still new. Several studies have been carried out to analyze the type of microbiota and many neurological diseases. Recently, changes in the microbiota have been linked to the onset of Parkinson's disease (PD). A current theory proposes PD as a disease that progresses parallel to the propagation of insoluble protein accumulations in the nervous system [30]. The enteric autonomic nervous system could be one of the starting points of this pathological accumulation of proteins, and a change in the microbiota that increases local inflammation and oxidative stress could initiate the pathological cascade, similar to what happens in experimental models. In addition, digestive autonomic changes, such as precocious constipation, are almost a preclinical constant in PD, and all this would support this hypothesis [31]. In certain neurological diseases, immunomodulatory drugs that seek to reestablish a situation in which the anti-inflammatory cytokines predominate in the system are used. The important relationship of the intestinal microbiota with the immune system offers the possibility of acting on the intestinal bacteria to achieve this change. Experimentally, and through this mechanism, treatment with certain antibiotics has influenced the prognosis of cerebral infarctions in experimental animals [32]. It is possible that the lack of knowledge about the etiopathogenesis of many neurological diseases and the gut microbiota prevents us from seeing the magnitude of the relationship between them and the possibilities of intervention to protect health or prevent or ameliorate diseases. Beyond the knowledge of all agents of the microbiota, their genes, and their functions, it is even more important to identify the molecules they produce and their effects on metabolism. Advances in proteomics and metabolomics with practical applications in the daily clinic may be the key to establishing microbiota profiles and the different relationships with neuronal diseases [33] (**Figure 6**).

4.1. Parkinson's disease

Recently, possible changes in the microbiota have been linked to the onset of Parkinson's disease (PD). A current theory suggests that PD is a disease that progresses parallel to the

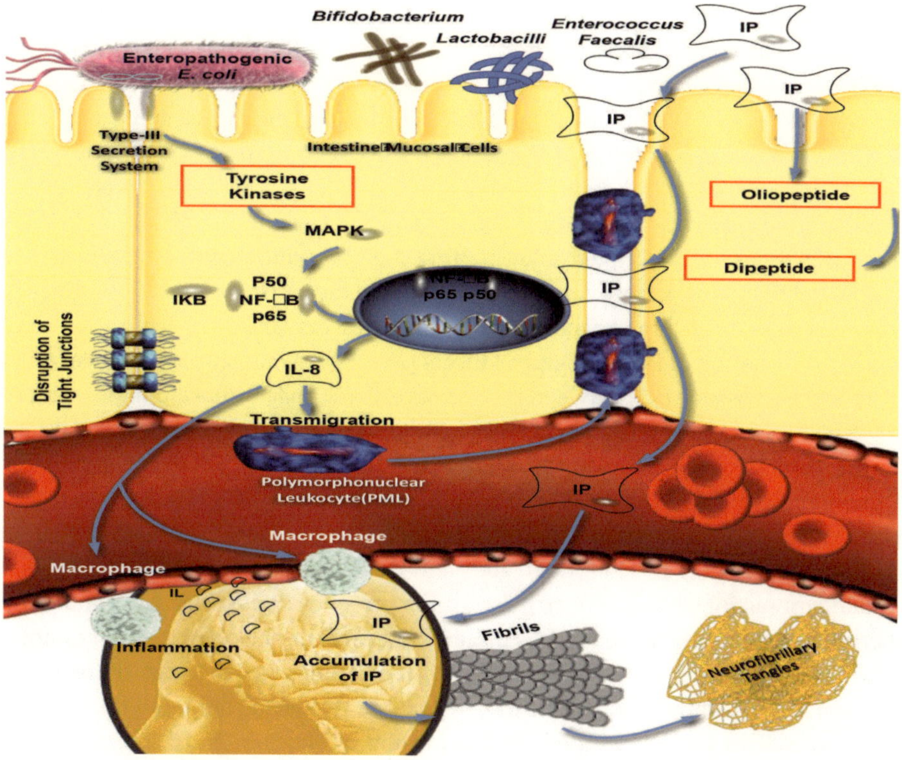

Figure 6. This figure shows the effect of the microbiota on the increased inflammation that results in Parkinson's disease. In addition, the accumulation of insoluble proteins may be an explanation for the pathological accumulation of proteins in the nervous system. IP, insoluble protein; NF-kB, nuclear factor kappa enhancer of activated B cells; MAPK, mitogen-activated protein kinase; P50, cytochromes P450; IKB, inhibitor of kB; IL-8, interleukin 8. This image is a modification of QIAGEN's original at www.QIAGEN.com/es/shop/genes-and-pathways/pathway-details/?pwid=29.

propagation of accumulations of insoluble proteins in the nervous system. The enteric autonomic nervous system could be one of the starting points of this protein accumulation. A change in the microbiota that increased local inflammation and oxidative stress could start the pathological cascade, similar to what happens in experimental models of PD. In addition, the autonomic changes to digestive disorders, such as precocious constipation, are almost a preclinical constant in PD, and all this would support this hypothesis [34]. In Parkinson's disease, a direct correlation between the amount of *Enterobacteriaceae* microbes in the gut of patients, and the degree of severity in the problems of balance and mobility was detected: Scheperjans explains that the abundance of *Enterobacteriaceae* was related to a high degree of postural instability and gait difficulty; therefore, there is a connection between the intestinal microbiota and the motor symptoms of our patients [35]. The question is, if the differences are permanent and whether the intestinal bacteria are linked to the progression of the disease and therefore to its prognosis. This fact implies that if we can establish the basis of the relationship between the intestinal microbiota and PD we will be in a much better position for developing new strategies for prevention of the disease and its progression [35, 36]. Microbial metabolites have been shown to influence the basic physiology of the blood-brain barrier. Intestinal microorganisms break down complex carbohydrates into short chains of fatty acids with a set of effects; for example, fatty butyric acid strengthens the blood-brain barrier by adjusting the connections between cells. Also, there are recent studies of neurotransmitters that could enable them to communicate with neurons. For example, it has been studied how certain metabolites of the bacterial microbiota promote the production of serotonin in the cells lining the colon, an interesting finding given that some antidepressant drugs work promoting serotonin at the junctions between neurons [37]. Even though the association of gastrointestinal disorders and PD has been studied extensively, it does not occur in the same way with the study of the influence of the gut microbiota on PD. The first studies in this regard were limited to evaluating the association between *Helicobacter pylori* infestation and PD. These investigations were based on the causal role of *H. pylori* in a variety of human diseases including chronic gastritis, peptic ulcers, and stomach cancer and in the well-known association of PD with gastric ulcers [38–41]. Several studies have demonstrated the existence of an association between PD and levels of *H. pylori* infestation. In a small, case-control study, a fivefold increase in *H. pylori* antibody levels was observed among patients older than 80 years of age with Parkinsonian manifestations [42]. Similarly, in patients with PD, a threefold increase in *H. pylori* antibody levels compared to control subjects has been reported. More recently, in an extensive study conducted in Denmark that included a total of 4484 PD patients diagnosed between 2001 and 2008, and a total of 22,416 controls, it was shown that chronic infections with *H. pylori* or the presence of gastritis contributed to PD or that there are pathologies related to this disease that precede the occurrence of motor symptoms. Additionally, it has been shown that the eradication of *H. pylori* infections decreases PD symptoms [43]. Composition of the *fecal microbiome* has been compared between patients with PD and control subjects in the District Hospital of Helsinki and Uusimaa [44]. In this study, 72 patients with idiopathic PD and an equal number of control individuals matched by sex and age were included. The existence of alterations of the intestinal microbiome in patients with PD was demonstrated, and such alterations were associated to the motor phenotype. The average abundance of the *Prevotellaceae* was reduced in 77.6% in the patients with PD in comparison with the control subjects. The relative abundance of *Prevotellaceae* of 6.5% or less had a sensitivity of 86.1% and a specificity of 38.9%, while a classifier obtained by logistic regression based on the abundance of four bacterial families and the severity of constipation identified PD patients with a sensitivity of 66.7% and a specificity of 90.3%. On the other hand, the relative abundance of *Enterobacteriaceae* was positively associated with the severity of postural instability and difficulty walking. The enterotype of the intestinal microbiota represented by *Prevotella* has been associated with increased levels of short-chain fatty acids with a neuroactive health-promoting function and with a high capacity for the synthesis of thiamine and folate. From these observations, it has been proposed that the observed decrease in the abundance of *Prevotella* could be associated to the previously reported decrease in the levels of these vitamins in PD patients and that the supplementation of these vitamins and short-chain fatty acids may have potential therapeutic effects in patients with PD.

4.2. Demyelinating diseases

There is a broad line of research on the relationship between intestinal microbiota and optic neuromyelitis and mainly with experimental autoimmune encephalomyelitis (EAE), an animal model of multiple sclerosis (MS), and an emerging line that is trying to extrapolate the results of the EAE to the MS. Patients with aquaporin-positive neuromyelitis optical have a higher serum antibody response to gastrointestinal antigens than healthy controls, especially in extensive myelitis, which seems to be related to the control of the microbiota on autoimmune inflammation [45]. The peripheral existence of aquaporin-specific T cells, capable of developing Th responses, which showed cross-reactivity with a homologous sequence in an epitope present in *Clostridium perfringens,* representative of the commensal flora, has also been demonstrated, insinuating a mechanism of responsible cellular mimicry of activating said Th response [46]. Demyelination usually occurs as a phenomenon secondary to an infectious disorder or a toxin. In the primary demyelinating processes, its cause is unknown, but an autoimmune mechanism is thought to occur because its appearance sometimes follows a virosis, an antiviral vaccination, or an alteration of the microbiota. Demyelination tends to be segmental or patchy and often affects multiple zones at once or in succession. Often remyelination occurs, with repair, regeneration, and complete recovery of nerve functions. However, any extensive loss of myelin is often followed by axonal degeneration and, often, also of cellular soma, and both processes can be irreversible. Demyelination should be considered for any patient suffering from a neurological deficit without any other explanation. Primary demyelinating disorders are suggested by:

- Diffuse or multifocal deficits
- Sudden onset, especially in young adults
- Appearance within weeks after an infection or vaccination
- A course with ups and downs
- Symptoms indicative of a specific demyelinating process (e.g., unexplained optic neuritis or internuclear ophthalmoplegia that suggests multiple sclerosis).

4.3. Multiple sclerosis

MS is caused by a combination of genetic and environmental factors. Among the causal factors, it could be that a certain individual with certain bacterial microbiota could more easily develop the disease. However, if we want to identify what happens with the gut microbiota, we might also include this within the environmental causes of the individual and understand the conditioning of the disease. The first line of work is to identify if the bacterial flora plays a role in multiple sclerosis and the second, if it plays a role, is to determine which bacteria are protective and which are harmful [21, 47]. This surprising finding was made possible by the recent development of genetically modified mice. In the absence of exposure to any external influences, inflammatory reactions emerge in the brains of these animals that are similar to those associated with multiple sclerosis in humans, yet this only occurs when mice have intact gut microbiota [48]. Mice without microorganisms in their gut, which remained in a sterile environment, remained healthy. When vaccinated, animals bred under sterile conditions, with normal intestinal microorganisms, also became ill; however, the gut microbiota influences the immune systems in the digestive tract, and mice without intestinal flora have fewer T cells. On the other hand, the spleen of these animals produces fewer inflammatory substances, like cytokines, and, in addition, B cells produce few or no antibodies against myelin and restore the microbiota of mice, and their T cells and B cells increase their production of cytokines and antibodies [49].

Another group of habitual commensal bacteria related to the regulation of the immune response and studied in EAE is lactic acid bacteria. Within this group is *Pediococcus acidilactici,* which is administered orally and induces an IL-10 mediated response that decreases the severity of EAE both therapeutically and prophylactically, through the inhibition of IL-17 and IFN-γ and a decrease in cellular infiltrates in the CNS. In this case, the responsible, related lymphocytes, rather than being TCD4 + FoxP3+ (with a slight increase), were the type 1 regulatory T lymphocytes (Treg1) [50]. The potential use of probiotics in EAE has been investigated. *Bifidobacterium animalis* has been used during lactation of rodents that were later induced for EAE, with a reduction in the duration of clinical symptoms, curiously only in male mice. Using a combination of three strains of *Lactobacillus,* they demonstrated that the combination, but not each separately, reversed EAE in mice, associated with an increase in TregFoxP3 + lymphocytes and IL-4, IL-10 and TGFβ1 in the nodules of lymphatic vessels and the spleen [50]. Using other mixtures of probiotics (*Lactobacillus, Bifidobacterium, and Streptococcus*), similar results have been obtained, as well as the association of IL-10 and the development of Treg in the mechanism, which, as previously mentioned, leads to a lower polarization of lymphocytes T helper toward Th1/Th1 [51]. Scientists would now like to analyze the total microbial genome of patients with multiple sclerosis and thus identify differences in the intestinal flora of healthy individuals and patients with multiple sclerosis. Scientists are sure that the microbiota can also trigger an exaggerated reaction of the immune system against the myelin layer in people with a genetic predisposition for multiple sclerosis. Therefore, nutrition can play a central role in the disease since diet largely determines the bacteria that colonize the intestine. Changing eating habits could explain, for example, why the incidence of multiple sclerosis has increased in Asian countries in recent years. Apparently the immune system is activated in two stages. First, the T cells in the lymphatic vessels of the gut are activated and proliferate together with the proteins of the surface of the myelin layer, and these stimulate the B cells to form pathogenic antibodies. Both processes trigger inflammatory reactions in the brain that progressively destroy the myelin layer, a process that is very similar to the way multiple sclerosis develops in humans [52]. How does the intestinal flora influence the health of the brain? This is an area that arouses more and more interest in those who work with neurodegenerative diseases, and understanding this balance and how to control it can open the way to a new type of probiotic-based therapy (foods that contain live bacteria that may be beneficial), synbiotics which stimulate the growth of existing beneficial bacteria (**Figure 7**).

In another study, it has been shown that there is a link between intestinal commensal bacteria and autoimmune pathologies in murine models of MS. In one study, 34 pairs of monozygotic twins were selected, one ill and the other not. This choice permits eliminating the influence of genetic factors and reducing the environmental factors in the appearance of MS. In advance, they compared fecal microbiota without finding important differences, except for an excess of *Akkermansia* in untreated sick subjects. To test the functionality of these intestinal floras, they selected five pairs of twins. The intestinal microbiota of each individual was transferred to rodents predisposed to autoimmune encephalomyelitis, which is the animal model of MS. This transplant triggered the disease in more than 60% of the animals that received microbiota from subjects with MS, compared to 30% in those who received the microbiota of healthy subjects. The analysis of the intestinal microbiota of the transplanted animals revealed an increase of the *Sutterella* deficit in the animals that received the microbiota of subjects with MS. However, the

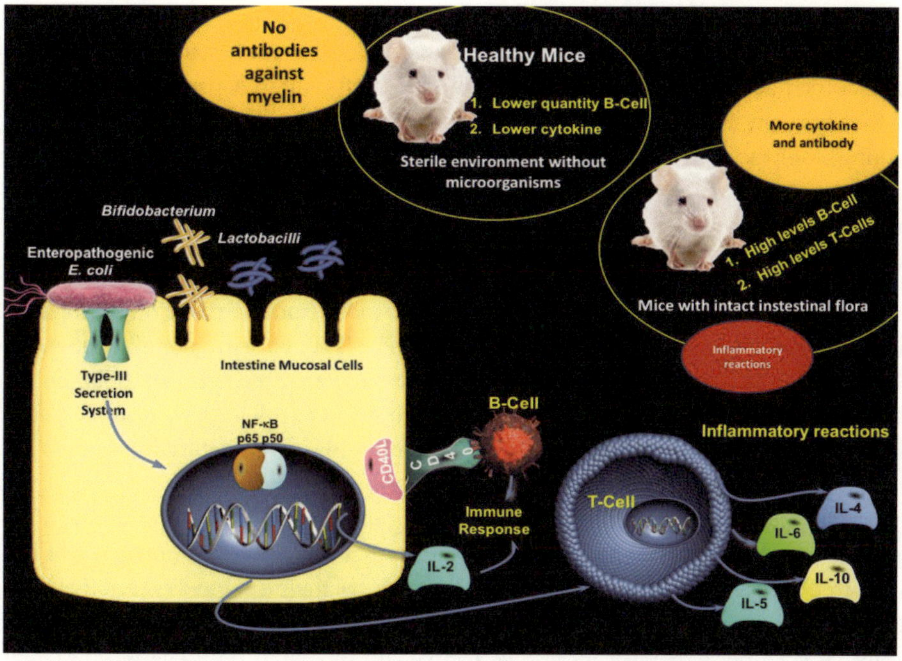

Figure 7. This figure shows an inflammatory pathway in mice very similar to that developed in MS patients. This inflammatory reaction is associated with modifications in the intestinal microbiota in mice. This image is a modification of QIAGEN's at www.QIAGEN.com/es/shop/genes-and-pathways/pathway-details/?pwid=29.

presence of this bacterium was associated with a better defense against inflammatory diseases. At the immune level, the study shows a deficit in the production of interleukin 10 in the animals that received the EM microbiota. In parallel, the blockade of this cytokine in rodents that received the healthy microbiota increased the incidence of autoimmune encephalomyelitis, which suggests that this molecule has a regulatory role in autoimmune diseases of the central nervous system [53].

5. Alteration in protein conformation: microbiota and nervous system

One of the problems that exist in common in several neurological diseases is alterations in the folding of proteins. It is the process by which the sequence of amino acids adopts a three-dimensional structure that constitutes its native form. In some proteins, in addition to the native and unfolding states, there are partially folded states known as intermediates. The concentration of proteins in the cytoplasm is high. Despite this, proteins in the native state are not normally added. On the other hand, the denatured state has a very short half-life. In this sense, various evidences strongly suggest that the aggregation is due to the specific association of non-native states. Several diseases that exhibit deposits of aggregated proteins have been associated with genetic factors, that is, point mutations in the protein that cause their aggregation. How do mutations facilitate aggregation? In physicochemical terms, mutations can alter the stability or speed of interconversion between the native form and the fibrillar form; denaturing conditions have been found that favor the presence of non-native conformations, which act as precursors of the formation of the altered proteins. Another coincidence that exists in several neuropathologies is that we know what is happening (not always everything), but the root cause, what or who initiates, is unknown; we mention that this is multifactorial and, in it, we cover part of our ignorance. A particular case is the stabilization of the folding of α-synuclein, which is involved in Parkinson's disease, dementia associated with Lewy bodies, and the variant of Alzheimer's disease also associated with Lewy bodies.

As mentioned above, a large number of proteins without homology, or not associated with diseases, present conformational structural alterations. If so, why are not all proteins added? And at this point is when we have the obligation to analyze these neuropathologies in a systemic way. Our body has taken thousands of years to perfect itself, and we often forget that the set of systems that make up our body is a unit and that this is in constant interaction between its organs and systems but also with the environment and other organisms that are part of it, including the microbiota, which is currently telling us how there are close dialogs between our gut and our nervous system and other systems in a constant back and forth of information in both directions. In most diseases described above, their diagnosis is another challenge because only if we are strict enough we will only say probable Parkinson's disease, and this will only be corroborated with its *postmortem* study, the same happens with Alzheimer's. When classifying these diseases, we reach another coincidence in most of them—sporadic or genetic—and their percentages between them are similar 85–90% vs. 15–10% (respectively). Where the genetic and the environment are usually variations of the same symphony, at the end of the day, the relationship between the nervous system and the microbiota of the gut is a fact that invites us to reflect on the individuality of the systems and the need for research in translational medicine.

Author details

Genaro Gabriel Ortiz[1*], Luis H. de Loera-Rodriguez[1], José A. Cruz-Serrano[2], Erandis D. Torres-Sánchez[3], Miriam A. Mora-Navarro[1], Daniela L. C. Delgado-Lara[1], Irma Gabriela Ortiz-Velázquez[1], Héctor González-Usigli[4], Oscar K. Bitzer-Quintero[5] and Mario Mireles Ramírez[4]

*Address all correspondence to: genarogabriel@yahoo.com

1 Laboratory of Mitochondria-Oxidative Stress and Pathology, Neurosciences Division, Western Biomedical Research Center, Mexican Social Security Institute, Guadalajara, Mexico

2 Kurago Biotek, Guadalajara, Mexico

3 Ciénega University Center, University of Guadalajara, Ocotlán, Mexico

4 Department of Neurology, UMAE-HE, National Occidental Medical Center, Mexican Social Security Institute, Guadalajara, México

5 Neuroimmunomodulation Laboratory, Neurosciences Division, Western Biomedical Research Center, Mexican Social Security Institute, Guadalajara, Mexico

References

[1] Koboziev I, Reinoso-Webb C, et al. Role of the enteric microbiota in intestinal homeostasis and inflammation. Free Radical Biology and Medicine. 2014;**68**:122-133

[2] Castillo-Álvarez F, March-Sola ME. Role of intestinal microbiota in the development of multiple sclerosis. Neurology. 2017;**32**(3):175-184

[3] Hollister Emiliy B, Chunxu G, Versalovic J. Compositional and functional features of the gastrointestinal microbiome and their effects on human health. Gastroenterology. 2014;**146**(6):1449-1458

[4] Chow J, Lee Melanie S, Shen Y, et al. Host bacterial symbiosis in health and disease. Advances in Immunology. 2010;**107**:243-274

[5] Dando S, Mackay-Sim A, Norton R, Currie B, et al. Pathogens penetrating the central nervous system: Infection pathways and the cellular and molecular mechanisms of invasion. Clinical Microbiology Reviews. 2014;**27**(4):691-726

[6] Nassif X, Bourdoulous S, Eugène E, Couraud PO. How do extracellular pathogens cross the blood-brain barrier? Trends in Microbiology. 2002;**10**(5):227-232

[7] Imani Fooladi A, Mahmoodzadeh Hosseini H, Reza Nourani M, Khani S, Moayed Alavian S. Probiotic as a novel treatment strategy against liver disease. Hepatitis Monthly. 2013;**13**(2):e7521

[8] Siddiqui A, Usmani RI, Anwer S, Afsar S. Guillain-Barre syndrome occurring after rabies vaccination. The Journal of the Pakistan Medical Association. 2005;**55**(2):87-88

[9] den Besten G, van Eunen K, Groen Albert K, Venema K, et al. The role of short-chain fatty acids in the interplay between diet, gut microbiota, and host energy metabolism. Journal of Lipid Research. 2013;**54**(9):2325-2340

[10] Matricon J, Barnich N, Ardid D. Immunopathogenesis of inflammatory bowel disease. Self Nonself. 2010;**1**(4):299-309

[11] Kuhn K, Stappenbec T. Peripheral education of the immune system by the colonic microbiota. Seminars in Immunology. 2013;**25**(5):364-369. DOI: 10.1016/j.smim.2013.10.002

[12] Macpherson A, Geuking M, McCoy K. Immune responses that adapt the intestinal mucosa to commensal intestinal bacteria. Immunology. 2005;**115**(2):153-162

[13] Belkaid Y, Hand T. Role of the microbiota in immunity and inflammation. Cell. 2014; **157**(1):121-141

[14] Wu H-J, Wu E. The role of gut microbiota in immune homeostasis and autoimmunity. Gut Microbes. 2012;**3**(1):4-14

[15] Kamada N, Núñez G. Role of the gut microbiota in the development and function of lymphoid cell. Journal of Immunology. 2013;**190**(4):1389-1395

[16] Troy E, Kasper D. Beneficial effects of *Bacteroides fragilis* polysaccharides on the immune system. Frontiers in Bioscience. 2010;**15**:25-34

[17] Nielsen OL, Olsen HG, Iburg T, Jensen HE, Leifsson PS, Agerholm JS, Skovgaard K. Cytokine and acute phase protein mRNA expression in liver tissue from pigs with severe sepsis caused by intravenous inoculation of *Staphylococcus aureus*. In 2010 Annual Meeting SLB & IEIIS: Abstracts; 2010

[18] Mawe G, Hoffman J. Serotonin signaling in the gastrointestinal tract. Nature Reviews. Gastroenterology & Hepatology. 2013;**10**(8):473-486

[19] Silver J, Schwab M, Popovich P. Central nervous system regenerative failure: Role of oligodendrocytes, astrocytes, and microglia. Cold Spring Harbor Perspectives in Biology. 2015;**7**(3): a020602. DOI:10.1101/cshperspect.a020602

[20] Lyte M, John Cryan F. Microbial Endocrinology: The MicrobiotaGut-Brain Axis in Health and Disease Springer New York. Abilene, TX, USA: Texas Tech University Health Sciences Center; 2014. p. 2014

[21] Lee-Phillips M. Gut reaction: Environmental effects on the human microbiota. Environmental Health Perspectives. 2009;**117**(5):A198-A205

[22] Rogers G, Keating D, Young R, Wong M, Licinio J, Wesselingh S. From gut dysbiosis to altered brain function and mental illness: Mechanisms and pathways. Molecular Psychiatry. 2016;**21**(6):738-748

[23] Wang Y, Kasper L. The role of microbiome in central nervous system disorders. Brain, Behavior, and Immunity. 2014;**38**:1-12

[24] Mazzoli R, Pessione E. The neuro-endocrinological role of microbial glutamate and GABA signaling. Frontiers in Microbiology. 2016;**7**:1934

[25] Carpenter S. The gut feeling. American Psychological Association. 2012;**43**(8):50-54

[26] Carabotti M, Scirocco A, Maselli M, Severi C. The gut-brain axis: Interactions between enteric microbiota, central and enteric nervous systems. Annals of Gastroenterology. 2015;**28**(2):203-209

[27] Young S. Acute tryptophan depletion in humans: A review of theoretical, practical and ethical aspects. Journal of Psychiatry & Neuroscience. 2013;**38**(5):294-305

[28] Dichter G, Damiano C, Allen J. Reward circuitry dysfunction in psychiatric and neurodevelopmental disorders and genetic syndromes: Animal models and clinical finding. Journal of Neurodevelopmental Disorders. 2012;**4**(1):19

[29] Sarkar A, Lehto S, Harty S, Dinan T, Cryan J, Burnet P. Psychobiotics and the manipulation of bacteria-gut-brain signals. Trends in Neurosciences. 2016;**39**(11):763-781

[30] Umbrello G, Esposito S. Microbiota and neurologic diseases: Potential effects of probiotics. Journal of Translational Medicine. 2016;**14**:298

[31] Mulak A, Bonaz B. Brain-gut-microbiota axis in Parkinson's disease. World Journal of Gastroenterology. 2015;**21**(37):10609-10620

[32] Plaza-Diaz J, Gomez-Llorente C, Fontana L, Gil A. Modulation of immunity and inflammatory gene expression in the gut, in inflammatory diseases of the gut and in the liver by probiotics. World Journal of Gastroenterology. 2014;**20**(42):15632-15649

[33] Chang R, Shoemaker R, Wang WA. Novel knowledge-driven systems biology approach for phenotype prediction upon genetic intervention. IEEE/ACM Transactions on Computational Biology and Bioinformatics. 2011;**8**(5):1170-1182

[34] Haroon E, Raison C, Miller A. Psychoneuroimmunology meets neuropsychopharmacology: Translational implications of the impact of inflammation on behavior. Neuropsychopharmacology. 2012;**37**(1):137-162

[35] Scheperjans F, Aho V, Pereira PA, Koskinen K, Paulin L, Pekkonen E, Haapaniemi E, Kaakkola S, Eerola-Rautio J, Pohja M, Kinnunen E, Murros K, Auvinen P. Gut microbiota are related to Parkinson's disease and clinical phenotype. Movement Disorders. 2015;**30**(3):350-358

[36] Mulak A, Bonaz B. Brain-gut-microbiota axis in Parkinson's disease. World Journal of Gastroenterology. 2015;**21**(37):10609-10620

[37] Conlon M, Bird A. The impact of diet and lifestyle on gut microbiota and human health. Nutrients. 2015;**7**(1):17-44

[38] Cersosimo MG, Raina GB, Pecci C, Pellene A, Calandra CR, Gutiérrez C, et al. Gastrointestinal manifestations in Parkinson's disease: Prevalence and occurrence before motor symptoms. Journal of Neurology. 2013;**260**:1332-1338

[39] Zlotnik Y, Balash Y, Korczyn AD, Giladi N, Gurevich T. Disorders of the oral cavity in Parkinson's disease and parkinsonian syndromes. Parkinsons Disease. 2015;**2015**:379-482

[40] Cereda E, Cilia R, Klersy C, Canesi M, Zecchinelli AL, Mariani CB, et al. Swallowing disturbances in Parkinson's disease: A multivariate analysis of contributing factors. Parkinsonism & Related Disorders. 2014;**20**:1382-1387

[41] Fasano A, Visanji NP, Liu LW, Lang AE, Pfeiffer RF. Gastrointestinal dysfunction in Parkinson's disease. Lancet Neurology. 2015;**14**(6):625-639

[42] Weller C, Charlett A, Oxlade NL. Role of chronic infection and inflammation in the gastrointestinal tract in the etiology and pathogenesis of idiopathic parkinsonism. Part 3: Predicted probability and gradients of severity of idiopathic parkinsonism based on *H. pylori* antibody profile. Helicobacter. 2005;**10**:288-297

[43] Nielsen HH, Qiu J, Friis S, Wermuth L, Ritz B. Treatment for helicobacter pylori infection and risk of Parkinson's disease in Denmark. European Journal of Neurology. 2012;**19**:864-869

[44] Scheperjans F, Aho V, Pereira PAB, Koskinen K, Paulin L, Pekkonen E, et al. Gut microbiota are related to Parkinson's disease and clinical phenotype. Movement Disorders. 2015;**30**(3):350-358

[45] Kim S-M, Kim S-J, Lee HJ, Kuroda H, Palace J, Fujihara K. Differential diagnosis of neuromyelitis optica spectrum disorders. Therapeutic Advances in Neurological Disorders. 2017;**10**(7):265-289

[46] Bradl M, Lassmann H. Experimental models of neuromyelitis optica. Brain Pathology. 2014;**24**(1):74-82

[47] Belkaid Y, Hand T. Role of the microbiota in immunity and inflammation – NCBI – NIH. Cell. 2014;**157**(1):121-141

[48] Denic A, Johnson A, Bieber A, Warrington A, Rodriguez M, Pirko I. The relevance of animal models in multiple sclerosis research. Pathophysiology. 2011;**18**(1)

[49] Belkaid Y, Hand T. Role of the microbiota in immunity and inflammation. Cell. 2014; **157**(1):121-141

[50] Thomé R, Moraes A, Bombeiro A, dos Santos Farias A, Francelin C, Alves da Costa T, Di Gangi R, Barbosa dos Santos L, Rodrigues de Oliveira A, Verinaud L. Chloroquine treatment enhances regulatory T cells and reduces the severity of experimental autoimmune encephalomyelitis. PLoS One. 2013;**8**(6):e65913. DOI:10.1371/journal.pone.0065913

[51] Taverniti V, Guglielmetti S. The immunomodulatory properties of probiotic microorganisms beyond their viability (ghost probiotics: Proposal of paraprobiotic concept). Genes & Nutrition. 2011;**6**(3):261-274

[52] Guglielmi G. Gut microbes could help trigger multiple sclerosis. Biology Brain & Behavior Health. 2017;**357**. http://www.sciencemag.org/news/2017/09/gut-microbes-could-help-trigger-multiple-sclerosis. DOI:10.1126/science.app9323

[53] Berer K et al. Gut microbiota from multiple sclerosis patients enables spontaneous autoimmune encephalomyelitis in mice. Proceedings of the National Academy of Sciences of the United States of America; 2017. Oct 3;**114**(40):10719-10724. pii: 201711233. DOI: 10.1073/pnas.1711233114

Chapter 3

Educational Implications of Spatial Memory

Michele Tine, Sophie Lenihan and Clara Batchelder

Additional information is available at the end of the chapter

http://dx.doi.org/10.5772/intechopen.79893

Abstract

Spatial memory is recruited during many classroom-based activities. As such, it is essential for both educators and students to understand how it operates in a classroom context. This chapter begins by providing a systematic overview of how spatial memory is used across a variety of academic domains including math, language arts, and science. It also reviews some of the typical characteristics of students who have relatively poor spatial memory abilities. Finally, it discusses how to best provide efficacious classroom support for these students. Taken together, it provides an accessible overview of the educational implications of spatial memory that educators and students can consider when trying to optimize learning in their classrooms.

Keywords: education, learning, academic achievement, teaching, memory

1. Introduction

Children spend a significant portion of their lives actively engaged in classroom activities designed to help them learn content, concepts, procedures, and skills. Many of these activities require the use of their spatial memory, yet many educators and students are not well versed in what spatial memory is or how it works. As evidenced in the other chapters in this book, spatial memory can be operationalized through a myriad of lenses. For the purpose of the current chapter, we will focus on spatial memory as it relates to the human ability to store spatial information in our minds for short periods of time and use that spatial information in our current thinking. In other words, spatial memory is the spatial workspace that students use in classrooms everyday. The amount of spatial information a student can hold and use in this workspace increases with age, but there are also individual differences in the amount of spatial information students of the same age can hold and use. Throughout this chapter we will refer to the upper limit of the amount of spatial information a student can hold and use at one point in time as spatial memory capacity.

Ample research highlights the central role a student's spatial memory capacity plays in his or her ability to succeed in school [1]. Considering this fact, this chapter aims to provide an overview of how spatial memory is used across academic domains, unpack characteristics of students who have small spatial memory capacities (relative to their peers), and outline evidence-based methods to support such students. Our hope is that this information can help position educators and students to optimize learning.

2. The role of spatial memory in academic learning

2.1. Math

Math content and, in turn, math pedagogy change substantially as a child progresses through school. Not surprisingly, the role spatial memory plays in math learning also evolves significantly throughout the course of schooling.

2.1.1. Preschool

The link between spatial memory and math achievement in preschool-age students has been well documented [2]. In fact, a preschooler's spatial memory capacity is among the best predictors of their performance on arithmetic problems [3] and having a small spatial memory capacity is associated with deficiencies in a preschooler's arithmetic abilities [4]. One reason for this link seems to be the critically important role spatial memory plays in linking number words with quantities under the Triple Code Model [5, 6]. More specifically, preschool students learn through explicit instruction that number words (e.g. seven) and symbols (e.g. 7) correspond to visual and spatial quantities (e.g. an image of seven tokens). With time they develop internal mental models that permanently link numbers words and symbols to their appropriate visual and spatial quantities. In doing so, they begin to categorize number words and symbols according to size [5, 6]. Then, preschoolers use these mental models to solve arithmetic problems by adding or subtracting spatially based 'token' representations to or from one another [4]. As you can imagine, the larger a preschoolers' spatial memory capacity, the more fluidly they can use their mental model to solve arithmetic problems [2]. The role spatial memory plays in how preschoolers solve arithmetic problems helps explains why they are more accurate when solving non-verbal arithmetic problems than verbal arithmetic problems [4].

2.1.2. Elementary school

Spatial memory continues to play a role in mathematical thinking when students enter elementary school, but its involvement begins to decrease as they age. In the first few years of elementary school, its role is still fairly central. There is a strong correlation between math ability and spatial memory capacity in first grade students; 7-year-old who have high overall math abilities also have large spatial memory capacities [2] and 7-year-old with low math performance perform worse on spatial memory tasks [1]. In fact, at this age, spatial memory capacity predicts more than 10% of ones math scores [2]. Furthermore, research shows that spatial interference severely impairs the ability of 6-year-old to solve arithmetic problems [1]. Taken together, this evidence suggests that in early elementary school, students still rely quite heavily on their spatial memory to do math.

However, as students continue on in elementary school, they shift towards using more verbal-based strategies to do math. It appears that this transition begins when students are about 8-year-old; spatial interference only slightly impairs the ability of 8-year-old to accurately complete math problems [1]. Keep in mind spatial interference significantly impaired the ability of 6-year-old to accurately complete math problems [1]. V*erbal* interference, however, causes severe impairment in 8-year-old math ability [1]. Corresponding, spatial memory predicts only 3% of 9 and 10 year olds' scores on math achievement tests, while it predicted 10% of the scores of 7-year-old [2]. And by age 10 or 11, spatial memory is no longer a statistically significant predictor of performance in addition, subtraction, or multiplication [7].

Multiple theories explain these age-related differences: a developmental theory, a novelty theory, and a domain specificity theory. The developmental theory purports that the age-related shift from spatial- to verbal-based strategies simply mirrors the developmental trajectories of spatial and verbal memory. Some suggest spatial memory develops earlier than verbal memory primarily because younger students are taught using spatial strategies, like finger counting [7]. The thought is that such spatial instruction early on may promote the development of spatial memory early on. Then, with age and the natural language development that comes with it, student's verbal memory development "catches up" allowing students to rely on more on their verbal memory. In addition, in about third grade, many schools actually begin to teach students to use explicit verbal strategies to solve math problems, like rote memorization (e.g., memorize that 8 times 7 is 56); this may in part explain when this is precisely the age we begin to see a diminishing role of spatial memory [3].

The novelty theory proposes that spatial memory is activated when *all* students, regardless of age, first learn a novel math skill [7]. Aligned with the novelty theory is data that shows spikes in the predictive power of spatial memory on math achievement each time a new subdomain of math is introduced [7]. For example, the predictive power of spatial memory in the subdomains of addition and subtraction spikes in first grade when these subjects are introduced, and then the predictive power decreases. There is a similar pattern among third graders; the spike in the predictive power of spatial memory on multiplication skills is dependent on the specific time a school introduces multiplication. The same goes for fourth graders with division [8]. It is worth noting that while the increases in the predictive power of spatial memory on multiplication and division exist, they are quite small [7]. Novelty theorists explain that this is because while students of all ages use their spatial memory when confronted with new and difficult math problems, older students more quickly develop verbal strategies for solving these types of problems [8].

Finally, the domain specificity theory proposes that spatial memory is associated with different math domains to different degrees [8]. For example, addition and subtraction may rely heavily on spatial memory because these problems are often solved by physical or visual manipulation, whereas multiplication and division may rely more on verbal memory because they are often solved by verbally memorized facts [8]. Empirical data offers some support for this theory; while spatial memory is associated with all math domains, the relationship between math achievement and spatial memory is indeed much stronger for addition and subtraction than it is for multiplication and division [8].

Ultimately, all theories highlight a general shift in the role spatial memory plays in math; in early elementary school its role is quite strong, but as students progress through elementary school its role lessens some.

2.1.3. Adolescence

The role of spatial memory on math does not disappear after elementary school, though. Aligned with the novelty theory, adolescents rely more on their verbal memory when solving math problems with which they are familiar, but they still seem to rely on their spatial ability as a back-up strategy when they encounter complex math problems [2, 3]. Other data corroborates that the role of spatial memory is not completely gone when students enter adolescence. For example, 14-year-old's spatial memory capacity is still significantly related to their standardized math scores [9]. Similarly, spatial memory at age 18 is positively correlated with performance on the math section of the SAT [10], and measures of mental rotation predict SAT math scores [11]. Furthermore, spatial memory in adolescence is a strong predictor of future success in math-related fields. Adolescents with greater spatial ability at age 13 are more likely to major in science, technology, engineering, or mathematics (STEM) in college and pursue a career in the STEM field [10]. In fact, more than 90% of people who have a PhD in a STEM-related field scored in the top quartile for spatial ability at age 11 [12]. So, despite the diminishing effect of spatial memory on math over time, it is important to note that its role does not seem to taper to nothing.

2.2. Language arts

2.2.1. Reading

Before considering the role spatial memory has on reading, it is essential to highlight that reading is a remarkably complex and dynamic process. Spatial memory is just one of many cognitive processes that work in concert when a child reads. Understanding this caveat, we will review what research tells us about the relationship between spatial memory and reading (1) achievement, (2) fluency, and (3) comprehension.

According to a meta-analysis of close to 300 studies, spatial memory can predict reading achievement in elementary, middle, and high school students [13]. In fact, spatial memory the best predictor of reading achievement of all the cognitive processes examined, which included auditory discrimination, auditory memory, auditory blending, auditory comprehension, visual discrimination, visual-motor integration, visual closure, visual association, visual–spatial relationship, and figure-ground discrimination [13]. Please note: the meta-analysis was not intended to be an exhaustive search of all the processes involved in reading; there are many processes related to reading that were not included that account for significantly more variance in reading ability than those included. However, when focusing in on this particular set of processes, the relative role of spatial memory is noteworthy [13].

Some evidence even suggests that spatial memory may plays a role in reading fluency, or the ability to read text quickly, accurately, and with appropriate prosody [14]. Verbal memory plays a larger role, of course [15, 16], but students with fluency reading disorders show reduced verbal *and* spatial memory capacities compared to typically developing readers. An understanding of the specific type of spatial memory that might be involved is still emerging, but it seems that it might have something to do with the ability to move visual material in the mind, as students with reading fluency disorders do equally well as those without reading disorders on tasks utilizing static spatial memory tasks that do not involve reading [17].

When we turn to reading comprehension, the evidence is somewhat clouded. There is a strong relationship between overall "working memory" (verbal and spatial memory taken together) and reading comprehension [16, 18]. Yet, studies that have attempted to determine the unique contribution of spatial memory compared to verbal memory have found little evidence that spatial memory contributes anything to reading comprehension *above and beyond* verbal memory. With that said, it is clear that students construct spatially-based mental models of situations described in text and update the models as they continue to read [19]. Importantly, student's ability to construct and update these spatial mental models is predictive of reading comprehension for elementary, middle, and high school students [19], a clear suggestion that some aspect of spatial memory *does* play a role.

2.2.2. Writing

There is also some evidence that links spatial memory to early writing ability. For example, researchers found that spatial memory accounts for a unique proportion of the variance in student's spelling and independent text writing skills in preschool and kindergarten, even when controlling for verbal memory [20]. As students age, the importance of verbal memory increases as they become more practiced writers and transcribers and can maintain more complex strings of sounds in their minds. But in the early stages of writing, the spatial memory appears to be in high demand as students practice producing novel visual representations of formerly solely auditory information [20].

2.3. Science

Most of the work exploring the ways in which students use spatial memory during science focuses on scientific thinking, as opposed to science test scores. And, indeed, spatial memory appears to be critical to a student's ability to think like a scientist. This makes sense when considering that a student who has superior spatial memory is able to create mental models of complex scientific ideas and then mentally manipulate those models, an ability necessary for scientific thinking [21]. For example, when a scientific theory that is initially presented in words or as an equation, it is often then mentally transformed into an abstract spatial representation, such as a graph or model. Moreover, the process of scientific investigation often involves reconciling a theory-based spatial model with a competing data-based spatial model. According to the Next Generation Science Standards, this type of scientific investigation is encouraged in simple formats in elementary school and quite complex formats in high school and college. And it is certainly a process career scientists use; researchers observed that scientists often use visualization to mentally manipulate models and modify theories when confronted with disconfirming data [22]. Clearly, the visualization and imagery components of spatial memory are necessary for scientific investigation.

It is not surprising then that ample evidence suggests spatial memory abilities can be used to predict later success in scientific fields [23–27]. Spatial memory is also predictive of scientific creativity [12, 21] and students who have superior spatial memory become expert engineers or physical scientists at much higher rates than those who do not have such abilities [12].

For these reasons many argue that spatial memory measures should be regularly administered as a way to identify future talent in scientific domains [28], especially considering the need to identify and nurture scientific and technical talent is a national priority [29, 30]. But despite the potential utility, spatial ability has not been used as a way to identify promising future scientist students, nor has it been incorporated into K-12 scientific curricula or instruction. Many researchers have noted this neglect and have noted that is especially surprising in today's globally competitive world [31]. Richard E. Snow expressed his perplexity when saying:

> *"There is good evidence that [spatial ability] relates to specialized achievements in fields such as architecture, dentistry, engineering, and medicine. Given this plus the longstanding anecdotal evidence on the role of visualization in scientific discovery,. .. it is incredible that there has been so little programmatic research on admissions testing in this domain* ([32], p. 136)."

Instead, verbal ability is most often used to determine an individual's suitability for a position that requires a college degree, such as a scientist or engineer, while spatial memory has been used to determine suitability for trade work, such as a technician or mechanic [33]. We hope this chapter can provide educators with a better understanding of the power of spatial memory and will, in turn, be in a position to use it to identify future talent.

3. Characteristics of students with poor spatial memory

Thus far we have outlined how spatial memory is an underlying cognitive process used across a variety of academic tasks, including math, language arts, and science. Considering this, it makes sense that students with poorly developed spatial memory might struggle in these academic areas, and there is plenty of literature to show that this is the case [34–37]. Evidence suggests poor or underdeveloped spatial memory is related to a host of general classroom behaviors, as well. Furthermore, there is data to suggest that particular demographic groups may develop spatial memory abilities at different rate than other demographic groups. To best position teachers to be able to effectively set all students up for success, we will outline these characteristics below.

3.1. Poor spatial memory and classroom behavior

Beyond academic achievement, students with poor *general* memory also tend to demonstrate a set of common classroom behaviors. Teachers of students with relatively weak general memory capacity typically judge (elementary school aged) students as highly inattentive and have having high levels of distractibility [38]. They are also described as often forgetting that they are currently doing and failing to remember instructions and, in turn, not being able to complete everyday classroom tasks [34]. They are not hyperactive, though. Instead, these students exhibit reserved behavior profiles and struggle the most with attention in large group activities led by the teacher [38]. Furthermore, poor general memory has shown to be associated with a lack of creativity in complex problem solving and poor self-monitoring of own work among older students [34, 38]. These studies, along with others, paint a picture of a student who has difficult time remaining on task and focused, which is a precursor to learning. Most studies on this topic have measured how spatial and verbal memory *taken together* (i.e., what most refer to as general working memory) impact classroom behavior. More research need be done to determine how these behavioral problems can be linked specifically to the spatial memory subcomponent, but it is clear that both spatial and verbal memory contribute to the behaviors [38].

3.2. Poor spatial memory and demographics

There is also some burgeoning evidence linking spatial memory profiles with demographic groups. Girls and boys are far more alike than different on most measures of intelligence and cognitive processing, but they do differ in spatial memory. Females have been found to underperform males on spatial memory tasks as early as preschool and through high school [39–41]. A variety of psychobiological factors contribute to these gender differences [39], but the differences seem malleable. As a result, the spatial gender difference has been the impetus for many interventions.

Neighborhood type seems to be another demographic characteristic that is associated with differences in spatial memory. Our own research measured the verbal and spatial memory abilities of students living in rural and urban poverty. The students living in rural poverty had significantly smaller spatial memory capacities compared to the students living in urban poverty [42]. Interestingly, this weakness was specific to spatial memory. The students living in rural poverty had larger verbal memory capacities than the students living in urban poverty [42]. This work indicates that there is some relationship between impoverished rural contexts and spatial memory development, although the specific environmental factors associated with the relationship are still under investigation.

Finally, additional evidence shows students with fetal alcohol syndrome (FAS) exhibit impaired spatial memory. Specifically, those with FAS consistently demonstrate constructional apraxia, in addition to a wider range of spatial deficits [43]. While this link has been documented for some time, further research needs to determine the antecedents and consequences among students with FAS.

There are a variety of psychobiological and environmental variables that impact spatial memory development of these demographic groups, as well as typically developing students. The current consensus is that some demographic groups, like those we mention, are exposed to variables that impede the development of spatial memory and/or not exposed to variables that promote its development. Clearly, it is essential that future research determine the psychobiological and environmental factors at play so intervention and prevention work can be effectively designed and implemented.

4. Interventions to support spatial memory weaknesses

Aligned with the notion that spatial memory is (1) malleable and (2) associated with educational success, much effort has gone into trying to determine how one can improve a student's spatial memory. The types of interventions that have been designed and/or tested can be categorized into two subtypes: training of spatial memory and classroom adjustments to reduce the required load.

4.1. Training of spatial memory

Uttal and colleagues performed a meta-analysis of more than 200 studies to investigate the magnitude, durability, and generalizability of training on spatial skills [44]. They concluded that training effects of spatial skills have a moderate effect (Hedges's g = 0.47), are stable over time, and transfer to other spatial tasks. From this, they highlight how a "spatially enriched education could pay substantial dividends" (p. 352).

Aligned with this conclusion, there is evidence of success for spatial interventions for young students that include the use of increased spatial language, maps and models, as well as jigsaw puzzles [45]. Additionally, early building block skills have been linked to spatial ability; Casey and Andrews developed a spatial intervention that uses storytelling and block building to increase spatial skills in young students, particularly spatial visualization and mental rotation [46]. Specially, a teacher reads aloud a story in which the characters instruct the students to build specific structures with blocks. The intervention was successful in improving the spatial skills of kindergarteners, and as a result Casey and Andrews suggest that structured block building should be included in classrooms to develop the spatial skills of students [46].

Block building can also be a successful tool to improve the spatial memory among older students. Eight-year-old who participated in a block building intervention performed better on mental rotation tasks and had increased activity in the parahippocampus, a brain region that is involved in spatial memory [47]. In addition, playing the computer game Tetris has been linked to increased mental rotation skills in 8-year-old; thus, computer-based interventions can be used in schools to improve students' spatial abilities [48]. Finally, adding spatially challenging activities to school classes can help improve the spatial skills of students [44]. High school students who were trained to use two and three dimensional representations in a physics course performed better on the spatially demanding task of reading a topography map [44].

4.2. Classroom adjustments to reduce required load

In addition to interventions, suggestions have been made about how teachers can make adjustments to their classrooms to reduce the load placed on students' spatial memories during any given activity, thereby allowing them to succeed. Gathercole and Alloway's eight-step approach is among the best known and it was designed to help teachers manage students' spatial memory load and reduce the disruptive effects that heavy spatial memory loads have on learning [49]. The first step of this approach is for teachers to recognize spatial memory weaknesses by monitoring students for errors including incomplete recall, failure to follow directions, place-keeping errors, and task abandonment [49]. The second step is to monitor students' spatial memory during classwork by asking students for the details of their classwork and what they intend to do next and the third step is for teachers to assess the spatial memory demands of classroom activities [49]. Step four encourages teachers to then reduce the spatial memory loads of classroom activities if the demands exceed the spatial memory capacities of students [49]. To do so, teachers shorten the number of items to be remembered; increase familiarity of information students need to remember; turning multi-step tasks into independent steps; and providing and encouraging the use of memory aids, such as number lines or printed notes [49]. The fifth step is for teachers to be conscious of processing demands that increase spatial loads [49], as students may have the spatial memory capacity to succeed in classroom activities, but simultaneous processing tasks may cause working memory failures [49]. The sixth step is for teachers to repeat important information often and encourage students to request the repetition of this information [49]. The seventh the seventh step is for teachers to encourage the use of memory aids like number lines, counting devices, Dictaphones, dictionaries, teacher notes, and wall charts can help reduce the processing demands and storage load of a classroom activity [49]. Finally, the eighth step is for teachers to help students develop memory-relieving strategies [49]. Importantly, Gathercole and Alloway claim teachers can reduce the memory load by following the aforementioned steps *without reducing* the amount of content taught and, in turn, learned [49].

4.3. Health and spatial memory

It is also worth mentioning that there are behavioral and medical conditions that can hurt one's memory abilities. For example, regular tobacco use decreases memory function because the overall amount of oxygen that the brain receives is reduced [50]. Sleep patterns are also related to our ability to consolidate and retrieve information from our memory; if one wakes up frequently in the night or gets less than the recommended amount of sleep for their age, consolidation and retrieval can be negatively impacted in the short term [51]. Nutrition is essential for overall brain function, as well, and ample research has shown that deficiencies in specific vitamins (i.e., B1, B12, and E) can negatively affect memory [52]. Considering, it is not surprising that work has explored if and how nutritional supplements can improve memory. While the work is young and large scale, longitudinal, methodologically sound studies on young healthy humans have not yet been completed, there are promising results from studies about the potential positive impact of a variety of supplements on memory including ginko biloba, omega-3 fish oil supplements, Huperzine A, the amino acid Acetyl-L-carnitine, Bacopa, and the hormone DHEA. [53]

5. Conclusion

In conclusion, let us consider Jane, an 8-year-old student. Despite her best efforts and those of her teachers, Jane struggles to keep up with the academic progress of her classmates. She is a hard worker and very well liked by her peers, but her math, reading, and science scores are in the lowest quartile of her class. Jane has started to become discouraged by the fact that she cannot seem to keep pace with her classmates. As a result, she is beginning to complain to her parents that she "doesn't like school" and "doesn't want to go to school." At the most recent parent teacher conference Jane's teacher brought up that Jane has a hard time following her instructions. What is important for teachers, parents, and students like Jane to understand is that it is possible that her current spatial memory capacity may be one of the underlying mechanisms that explain her struggles. Fortunately, Jane's teachers can make the aforementioned classroom adjustments to lower that spatial load of classroom activities for Jane in ways that will not reduce learning. Simultaneously, research suggests that Jane may benefit from some training in spatial memory strategies. Jane should also consider her current health and behavioral tendencies, such as sleep and nutrition. Also, perhaps most importantly, if Jane is able to identify and understand the underlying cause of her difficulties, she may feel less discouraged and more hopeful as she continues though her education.

Author details

Michele Tine*, Sophie Lenihan and Clara Batchelder

*Address all correspondence to: michele.tine@dartmouth.edu

Dartmouth College, Hanover, New Hampshire, USA

References

[1] Pickering SJ, editor. Working Memory and Education. Amsterdam: Elsevier; 2006

[2] Holmes J, Adams J, Hamilton C. The relationship between visuospatial sketchpad capacity and children's mathematical skills. European Journal of Cognitive Psychology. 2008; **20**(2):272-289. DOI: 10.1080/09541440701612702

[3] Raghubar KP, Barnes MA, Hecht SA. Working memory and mathematics: A review. Learning & Individual Differences. 2010;**20**:110-122. DOI: 10.1016/j.lindif.2009.10.005

[4] Rasmussen C, Bisanz J. Representation and working memory in early arithmetic. Journal of Experimental Child Psychology. 2005;**91**:137-157. DOI: 10.1016/j.jecp.2005.01.004

[5] Krajewski K, Schneider W. Exploring the impact of phonological awareness, visual-spatial working memory, and preschool quantity-number competencies on mathematics achievement in elementary school: Findings from a 3-year longitudinal study. Journal of Experimental Child Psychology. 2009;**103**(4):516-530. DOI: 10.1016/j.jecp.2009.03.009

[6] Dehaene S, Cohen L. Towards an anatomical and functional model of number processing. Mathematical Cognition. 1995;**1**(1):83-120

[7] van der Ven SHG, van der Maas HLJ, Straatemeier M, Jansen BRJ. Visuospatial working memory and mathematical ability at different ages throughout primary school. Learning and Individual Differences. 2013;**27**:182-192. DOI: 10.1016/j.lindif.2013.09.003

[8] Van de Weijer-Bergsma E, Kroesbergen E, Van Luit JEH. Verbal and visual-spatial working memory and mathematical ability in different domains throughout primary school. Memory and Cognition. 2015;**43**(3):367-378. DOI: 10.3758/s13421-014-0480-4

[9] Gathercole SE, Pickering SJ, Knight C, Stegmann Z. Working memory skills and educational attainment: Evidence from national curriculum assessments at 7 and 14 years of age. Applied Cognitive Psychology. 2004;**18**(1):1-16. DOI: 10.1002/acp.934

[10] Tosto MG, Hanscombe KB, Haworth CMA, Davis OSP, Petrill SA, Dale PS, Malykh S, Pomin R, Kovas Y. Why do spatial abilities predict mathematical performance? Developmental Science. 2014;**17**(3):642-470. DOI: 10.1111/desc.12138

[11] Casey MB, Nuttall RL, Pezaris E. Mediators of gender differences in mathematics college entrance test scores: A comparison of spatial skills with internalized beliefs and anxieties. Developmental Psychology. 1997;**33**(4):669-680. DOI: 10.1037//0012-1649.33.4.669

[12] Wai J, Lubinski D, Benbow CP. Spatial ability for STEM domains: Aligning over 50 years of cumulative psychological knowledge solidifies its importance. Journal of Educational Psychology. 2009;**101**(4):817-835. DOI: 10.1037/a0016127

[13] Kavale KA, Forness SR. Auditory and visual perception processes and reading ability: A quantitative reanalysis and historical reinterpretation. Learning Disability Quarterly. 2000;**23**:253-270. DOI: 10.2307/1511348

[14] Hudson RF, Pullen PC, Lane HB, Torgesen JK. The complex nature of reading fluency: A multidimensional view. Reading and Writing Quarterly. 2009;**25**:4-32. DOI: 10.1080/10573560802491208

[15] Fischback A, Könen T, Rietz CS, Hasselhorn M. What is not working in working memory of children with literacy disorders? Evidence from a three-year longitudinal study. Reading and Writing: An Interdisciplinary Journal. 2014;**27**(2):267-286. DOI: 10.1007/s11145-013-9444-5

[16] Oakhill J, Yuill N, Garnham A. The differential relations between verbal, numerical and spatial working memory abilities and children's reading comprehension. International Electronic Journal of Elementary Education. 2011;**4**(1):83-106

[17] von Károlyi C, Winner E, Gray W, Sherman GF. Dyslexia linked to talent: Global visual-spatial ability. Brain and Language. 2003;**85**(3):427-431. DOI: 10.1016/S0093-934X(03)00052-X

[18] Nation K, Adams JW, Bowyer-Crane CA, Snowling MJ. Working memory deficits in poor comprehenders reflect underlying language impairments. Journal of Experimental Child Psychology. 1999;**73**:139-158. DOI: 10.1006/jecp.1999.2498

[19] Barnes MC, Raghubar KP, Faulkner H, Denton C. The construction of visual–spatial situation models in children's reading and their relation to reading comprehension. Journal of Experimental Child Psychology. 2014;**119**:101-111. DOI: 10.1016/j.jecp.2013.10.011

[20] Bourke L, Davies SJ, Sumner E, Green C. Individual differences in the development of early writing skills: Testing the unique contribution of visuospatial working memory.

Reading and Writing: An Interdisciplinary Journal. 2014;**27**(2):315-335. DOI: 10.1007/s11145-013-9446-3

[21] Trickett SB, Trafton JG. What if…: The use of conceptual simulations in scientific reasoning. Cognitive Science. 2007;**31**:843-375. DOI: 10.1080/03640210701530771

[22] Trafton JG, Trickett SB, Mintz FE. Connecting internal and external representations: Spatial transformations of scientific visualizations. Foundations of Science. 2005;**10**:89-106. DOI: 10.1007/s10699-005-3007-4

[23] Gohm CL, Humphreys LG, Yao G. Underachievement among spatially gifted students. American Educational Research Journal. 1998;**35**:515-531. DOI: 10.2307/1163447

[24] Humphreys LG, Lubinski D, Yao G. Utility of predicting group membership and the role of spatial visualization in becoming an engineer, physical scientist, or artist. Journal of Applied Psychology. 1993;**78**:250-261. DOI: 10.1037/0021-9010.78.2.250

[25] Lohman DF. Spatial abilities as traits, processes, and knowledge. In: Sternberg RJ, editor. Advances in the Psychology of Human Intelligence. Vol. 4. Hillsdale, NJ: Erlbaum; 1988. pp. 181-248

[26] Lohman DF. Spatial ability. In: Sternberg RJ, editor. Encyclopedia of Intelligence. Vol. 2. New York: Macmillan; 1994. pp. 1000-1007

[27] Lohman DF. Spatially gifted, verbally, inconvenienced. In: Colangelo N, Assouline SG, Ambroson DL, editors. Talent Development. Vol. 2. Proceedings from the 1993 Henry B. and Jocelyn Wallace National Research Symposium on Talent Development. Dayton, OH: Ohio Psychology Press; 1994. pp. 251-264

[28] National Science Board. Preparing the Next Generation of STEM Innovators: Identifying and Developing our Nation's Human Capital. 2010. Available from: http://www.nsf.gov/nsb/publications/2010/nsb1033.pdf

[29] American Competitiveness Initiative. American Competitiveness Initiative: Leading the World in Innovation. Washington, DC: Domestic Policy Council Office of Science and Technology; 2006

[30] National Academy of Sciences. Rising above the Gathering Storm. Washington, DC: National Academy Press; 2005

[31] Friedman TL. The World Is Flat: A Brief History of the Twenty-First Century. New York: Farrar, Straus & Giroux; 2005

[32] Snow RE. Commentary: Expanding the breadth and depth of admissions testing. In: Messick S, editor. Assessment in Higher Education. Hillsdale, NJ: Erlbaum; 1999. pp. 133-140

[33] Eliot J, Macfarlane SI. An International Directory of Spatial Tests. Windsor Berks, England: Nfer-Nelson; 1983

[34] Alloway TP. How does working memory work in the classroom? Educational Research and Reviews. 2006;**1**(4):134-139

[35] Berg DH. Cognitive impairments of children with severe arithmetic difficulties: Cognitive deficit or developmental lag? Exceptionality Education International. 2008;**18**: 59-92

[36] Mammarella IC, Lucangeli D, Cornoldi C. Spatial working memory and arithmetic deficits in children with nonverbal learning difficulties. Journal of Learning Disabilities. 2010;**43**(5):455-468. DOI: 10.1177/0022219409355482

[37] Toll SWM, Kroesbergen EH, Van Luit JEH. Visual working memory and number sense: Testing the double deficit hypothesis in mathematics. British Journal of Educational Psychology. 2016;**86**:429-445. DOI: 10.1111/bjep.12116

[38] Gathercole SE, Alloway TP, Kirkwood HJ, Elliott JG, Holmes J, Hilton KA. Attentional and executive function behaviours in children with poor working memory. Learning and Individual Differences. 2008;**18**:214-223. DOI: 10.1016/j.lindif.2007.10.003

[39] Reilly D, Neumann DL, Andrews G. Gender differences in spatial ability: Implications for STEM education and approaches to reducing the gender gap for parents and educators. In: Khine MS, editor. Visual-Spatial Ability: Transforming Research into Practice. Switzerland: Springer International; 2017. pp. 195-224. DOI: 10.1007/978-3-319-44385-0_10

[40] Linn MC, Petersen AC. Emergence and characterization of sex differences in spatial ability: A meta-analysis. Child Development. 1985;**56**(6):1479-1498. DOI: 10.2307/1130467

[41] Voyer D, Voyer S, Bryden MP. Magnitude of sex differences in spatial abilities: A meta-analysis and consideration of critical variables. Psychological Bulletin. 1995;**117**(2): 250-270. DOI: 10.1037//0033-2909.117.2.250

[42] Tine M. Working memory differences between children living in rural and urban poverty. Journal of Cognition and Development. 2014;**15**(4):599-613. DOI: 10.1080/15248372.2013.797906

[43] Uecker A, Nadel L. Spatial locations gone awry: Object and spatial memory deficits in children with fetal alcohol syndrome. Neuropsychologia. 1996;**34**(3):209-223. DOI: 10.1016/0028-3932(95)00096-8

[44] Uttal DH, Newcombe N, Meadow N. The malleability of spatial skills: A meta-analysis of training studies. Psychological Bulletin. 2013;**139**(2):352-402. DOI: 10.1037/a0028446

[45] Newcombe NS. Picture this: Increasing math and science learning by improving spatial thinking. American Educator. 2010;**34**(2):29-35

[46] Casey BM, Andrews N, Schindler H, Kersh JE, Samper A, Copley J. The development of spatial skills through interventions involving block building activities. Cognition and Instruction. 2008;**26**:269-309. DOI: 10.1080/07370000802177177

[47] Newman SD, Hansen MT, Gutierrez A. An fMRI study of the impact of block building and board games on spatial ability. Frontiers in Psychology. 2016;**7**:1278. DOI: 10.3389/fpsyg.2016.01278

[48] De Lisi R, Wolford JL. Improving children's mental rotation accuracy with computer game playing. Journal of Genetic Psychology. 2002;**163**:272-282. DOI: 10.1080/00221320209598683

[49] Gathercole SE, Alloway TP. Understanding Working Memory: A Classroom Guide. London: Hartcourt Assessment; 2007

[50] Ernst M, Matochick JA, Heishman SJ, Van Horn JD, Jons PH, Henningfield JE, London ED. Effect of nicotine on brain activation during performance of a working memory task. Proceedings of the National Academic of Sciences of the United States of America. 2001;**98**(8):4728-4733. DOI: 10.1073/pnas.061369098

[51] Maquet P. The role of sleep in learning and memory. Science. 2001;**294**(5544):1048-1052. DOI: 10.1126/sciecne.1062856

[52] Zemplenji J, Suittie JW, Gregory JF, Patrick J. Handbook of Vitamins. Hoboken, NJ: CRC Press; 2014

[53] Stuart A. Fortifying Your Memory with Supplements. Web MD. 2018. Available from: https://www.webmd.com/diet/features/fortifying-your-memory-with-supplements#1

Chapter 4

True and False Memories: Neuropsychological and Neuropharmacological Approaches

Regina Vieira Guarnieri,
Orlando Francisco Amodeo Bueno and
Ivanda de Souza Silva Tudesco

Additional information is available at the end of the chapter

http://dx.doi.org/10.5772/intechopen.80918

Abstract

Some recent studies have explored the false memory and its mechanisms. True memories depend on draw in the past, retrieve of the information, remember past events plus recombine (reorganize) them with new information to finally re-encode these elements creating a new memory. But, sometimes failures in this system lead to memory errors collaborating to false memory formation. This chapter will address new neuropsychological tools to evaluate true and false memory performance. Some neuropharmacological aspects as possible mechanisms of agonist and antagonist modulation of false memory will be discussed.

Keywords: false memory, episodic memory, neuropsychology, neuropharmacology

1. Introduction

1.1. Memory

Memory can be described as the ability to acquire and retain new information and retrieve it in a conscious or unconscious way when necessary, being composed of a set of independent systems acting in a cooperative way [1]. Daily, we perform several numbers of tasks, such as reading a newspaper, calculating the tip at the restaurant, imagining a new layout of the furniture in our living room to fit a new sofa, comparing qualities and defects of apartments to choose the one that we will rent, and so on. Finally, tasks involving multiple steps that need to be kept mentally until a result is established [2].

1.2. Types of memory: short-term memory, working memory, and long-term memory

Memory is, in theory, fragmented into short-term memory, working memory, and long-term memory.

In 1890, James was the first one to propose the separation of memory in two systems: the primary memory, which nowadays could be equivalent to the concept of working memory, and the secondary memory that would be analogous to the long-term memory [3]. Atkinson and Shiffrin [4] proposed the model known as a modal model that would process information at three interconnected levels: (1) modal sensory register, (2) short-term memory, and (3) long-term memory, the latter being understood as a permanent storage of information (**Figure 1**). According to this model, information from external environmental stimuli are processed in different parallel sensorial registers, being stored in a short-term system (primary) with limited capacity and later in long-term memory (secondary). In this model, the role of short-term storage is crucial to achieve long-term storage, as well as to the retrieval of information contained in this system. The concept of short-term memory refers to the ability to process and store a few items, about four, for a very short period (seconds) decaying rapidly over time [5]. Despite this rapid forgetting rate, information can be kept longer in memory through rehearsal [4].

One of the most influential models of working memory is that of Baddeley and Hitch proposed in 1974 [6]. The model postulates two processing and manipulation loops: the phonological loop capable of maintaining and processing verbal information and the visuospatial sketchpad which similarly handles visual information. In addition, there is one more attentional component, the central executive, who coordinates all information from these subsystems. More recently, another integrator component has been incorporated into the model; the episodic buffer where information is temporarily held and manipulated before being definitively stored in long-term memory. The episodic buffer is a limited capacity storage system that temporarily keeps information under the control of the central executive [7]. Working memory is important in focusing attention, logic, reasoning, planning, strategy, and learning processes (**Figure 2**) [8].

Long-term memory is defined as the ability of the subject to acquire, retain, and retrieve information from events that occurred hours, days, months, or even years ago. According to Squire and

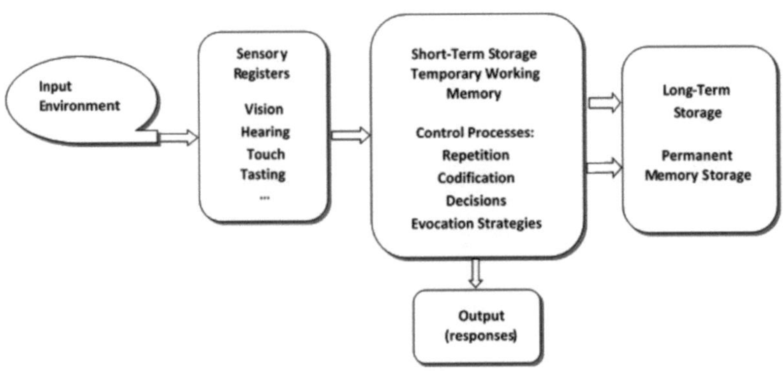

Figure 1. Modal model adapted from Atkinson and Shiffrin [4].

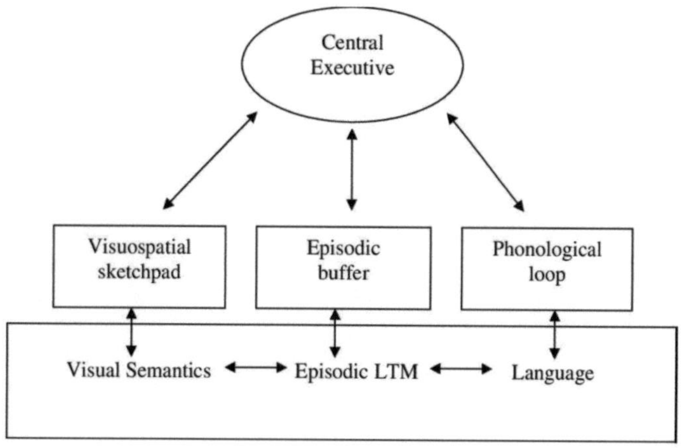

Figure 2. Model of working memory adapted from Baddeley.

Zola-Morgan [9], long-term memory can be subdivided into declarative (or explicit) memory and non-declarative (or implicit) memory. Explicit memory refers to the ability to store and consciously remember facts and events; otherwise, the implicit memory is independent of consciousness or intentional recollection and concerns learning, motor, and cognitive skills acquired gradually. Most memories stored in implicit memory are procedural memories. It involves several types of cognitive abilities, which can be measured through the performance of the individual. It occurs through the learning of a series of habits and abilities, making it easier to remember after exposure to specific stimuli, such as priming, classical and operant conditioning, and nonassociative learning [10].

Declarative memory depends on the integrity of medial temporal lobe structures including the hippocampus, parahippocampal gyrus, entorhinal and perirhinal cortices, fornix, and anterior and mediodorsal nuclei in the thalamus. Particularly, it is primarily dependent on mesial temporal lobe structures, especially the hippocampus [9]. Declarative memory is conceptually subdivided into semantic memory and episodic memory. The semantic memory is relative to the ability to acquire knowledge in general, such as knowledge of the world, concepts, and vocabulary, and does not depend on context for its evocation [11]. Episodic memory is a type of declarative memory that temporarily receives and stores information and its temporospatial relationships.

The episodic memory is the one who is most interested in the studies of false memories. Retrieval, also known as recall or remembering, is considered the reaccessing of events or information previously encoded and stored in our brain in the past. On the other hand, recognition is a subcategory of declarative memory, defined as the ability to recognize previously encountered events, objects, or people.

To test false memory, one can apply the word free recall task on subjects because it implies the recall of some words on a given occasion, that is, within a certain temporospatial context, but also recognition task is verily applied in several studies related to this topic (see items 2 and 3) (**Figure 3**).

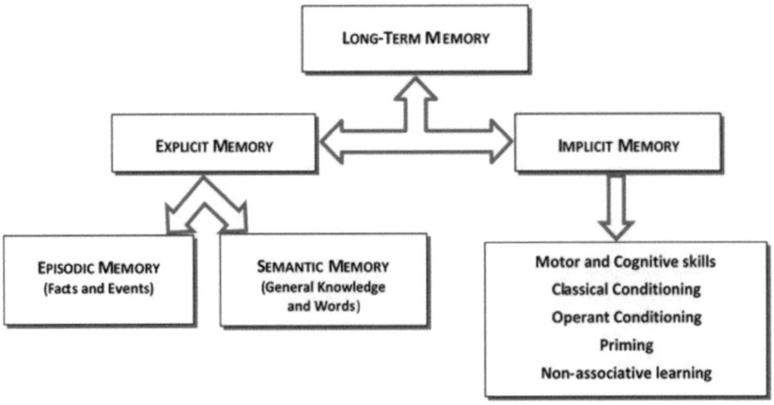

Figure 3. Long-term memory according to Squire and Zola's [9] definition.

So far, we have explored the types of memory: short-term memory, long-term memory, and working memory, which also clearly play a role in false memory processes. Now, we will present a very important type of memory in the formation of false memories, which is the emotional memory.

1.3. Emotional memory

Emotional reactions can be measured according to subjective reports (e.g., evaluation scales), objectives (e.g., physiological responses, such as heart rate and electrical conductance), and observation of behaviors (e.g., expressions) [12].

Human emotional experiences can be characterized by two main affective dimensions: valence and arousal. Valence refers to a continuous evaluation that varies from unpleasure (negative valence-unpleasant) to pleasure (positive valence-pleasant), passing through the neutral classification. The arousal refers to a continuous evaluation that varies from calm to stimulation. The emotional reaction to any stimulus (e.g., images and words) can be classified according to the valence and the arousal. In 1980, Lang developed a nonverbal pictographic measure for the subjective evaluation of valence and the arousal, the Self-Assessment Manikin (SAM) [13]. The SAM has the purpose of evaluating more objectively the affective dimensions of stimuli, used in studies on motivation, attention, and memory. At this task, usually, a stimulus that causes emotional reactions with low levels of valence is classified as negative, with medium levels as neutral, and with high levels as positive. Likewise, for the arousal, low-level stimuli are described as relaxing, with medium levels as non-stimulating and with high levels such as arousal.

Words and photographs classified as being of negative or positive valence present stimulating arousal level and are more likely to be correctly retrieved than similar stimuli classified as neutral and not stimulant [14]. Additionally, some studies have suggested that the arousal reinforces the encoding of central aspects of a stimulus through unintentional attention mechanisms while at the same time tends to decrease the encoding of peripheral details of stimuli [15]. For example, looking at a photo of an accident between two cars on a highway, people tend to remember more the central and significant aspects of the event (e.g., crumpled cars) than the peripheral aspects of the event (e.g., a traffic board or advertisement billboards on the side of the road) [16]. Sometimes these circumstances facilitate the false memory formation once some peripheric details could not be well encoded and may be re-encoded in a wrong way and falsely retrieved in the future.

Several studies have shown that episodes that contain emotional relevance have a greater probability of being remembered than those that do not contain it: so, there are advantages in the retrieval of stimuli classified as stimulants compared to non-stimulating stimuli. The emotion promotes better encoding of the memory trace due to greater rehearsal, attention, and elaboration that it provides [17].

The amygdala is the primary orchestrator of emotional memory without which the emotional effects in memory do not occur. The amygdala is responsible for the incremental effect of emotion in declarative memory [18]. The amygdala affects the memory, whether in encoding as in storage, modulating, or increasing the activity of other brain regions, such as the hippocampus. On the other hand, the hippocampus influences the responses of the amygdala when emotional stimuli are involved [19]. A case study of a patient who had bilateral lesion of the amygdala related that he did not enjoy the typical benefit of emotion in increasing the memory for images of positive or negative emotional content [20]. Another interesting data come from a functional magnetic resonance study dependent on the blood oxygenation-level-dependent functional magnetic resonance imaging (BOLD fMRI)reporting that Parkinson's patients present abnormal activation of the amygdala that is associated with deficiencies in responses to emotional stimuli of fear [21].

There are two main effects of emotion in explicit memory, both mediated by the amygdala: *effect at the time of encoding*, including increased attention and elaboration, and the post-encoding effect that includes the release of cortisol and increased consolidation of memory trace. *At the time of memory consolidation*, the hormones released in the hypothalamus-pituitary-adrenal axis, under the influence of the amygdala, act in the hippocampus assisting the storage of stimuli, making them more resistant to forgetting and interference. In this way, it facilitates retrieval [22].

Emotional valence can affect explicit memory through its influence on the activity of the adeno-pituitary gland, modifying the release of stress hormones that interact with the amygdala. The modulation effect of emotional valence, through the amygdala action, acts specifically in the areas of memory consolidation such as the hippocampus. Studies have shown that the amygdala and hippocampus systems are independent. For example, one of these studies used the fear-conditioning paradigm where the emergence of a blue square on the screen is halted with a shock to the wrist. Patients with amygdala lesions did not show the normal physiological response of fear of dodging the shock, although they reported that they knew that the blue square preceded the same. That is, the prediction of what was going to occur, that is, the event itself, was intact, because it depends on the hippocampus, while the emotional link does not. Patients with damage to the hippocampus showed an opposite pattern [23]. There is evidence that the activation of the amygdala can be modulated by attention. The amygdala does not respond differently to faces with emotional content when attentional resources are being divided to another focus, which indicates that the emotional processing in the amygdala is susceptible to "top-down" control [24].

Other important anatomical areas activated during emotional memory processing are the anterior cingulate cortex, nucleus accumbens, septum, ventral tegmental area, insula, somatosensory cortex, and brainstem. A study of functional neuroimaging demonstrated a correlation between the activation of the anterior cingulate cortex, emotion, and attention [25]. In 2000, Bush and collaborators published a review that cites several studies that evidence the involvement of the anterior cingulate cortex in a circuit involving attention in the regulation of cognitive and emotional processes [26]. Evidence suggests that this area is activated during the perception of emotion, affection, and pain, during the symptoms of post-traumatic disorder and the detection of errors [26, 27]. The anterior cingulate cortex is, in turn, related to the visceral, attentional, and emotional integration of the information involved with the regulation of affection and other forms of "top-down" control. It is also suggested that it is the key substrate for emotional awareness and the central representation of the autonomic arousal. These neuroimaging studies involving various types of emotional stimuli have determined the affective subdivision of the anterior cingulate cortex. It seems that this area is activated when the subject must monitor conflicts between the functional state of the organism and any new information that has relevant affective and emotional consequences. When such conflicts are detected, the areas of the anterior cingulate cortex project to the prefrontal cortex and nuclei of the base where options for responses will be evaluated. The prefrontal cortex plays an important role in emotion feedback; particularly, the ventromedial prefrontal cortex is active when decisions need to be made based on the emotional properties of the stimuli [30]. Generally, behavioral choices that require decision-making are influenced by the immediate affective consequence of a situation (e.g., a reward). In these situations, regions of the left prefrontal cortex are active when the target is related to appetitive situations, while the right prefrontal cortex is activated in negative [28, 29].

2. False memory

True memory is the real retrieval of an event of any nature, be it visual, verbal, or otherwise. True memories are constantly being rewritten (re-encoding). On the other hand, false memory is defined as the recollection of an event that did not happen or a distortion of an event that indeed occurred. Otherwise, confabulation is the formation of false memories, perceptions, or beliefs about yourself or the environment because of neurological or psychological dysfunction. During this process, confusion between imagination and memory or even confusion between true memories may occur.

Since the past decade, the phenomenon of false memories is drawing attention in the mental health area. Research in the field of mental health and legal area has suggested that emotion can influence the production of false memories. Some studies have indicated that certain psychotherapeutic techniques which are based on the retrieval of emotional memories in children can produce vivid memories of events that have not really occurred, for example, alleged cases of sexual violence suffered during childhood [30]. The memory of these children can be reconfigured in the wrong way. In the legal area, the impact of emotion on the functioning of memory may compromise the exercise of justice, since the person who has witnessed some crime, violation, and/or suffer if any kind of violence may be subject to distortion of their memories [31].

The relationship between the emotion and the production of false memories, however, is difficult to test with autobiographical memories since a detailed comparison between the information retrieved and details of the original event is practically unfeasible [16, 32].

False memories can also occur in the ordinary day-to-day life (not necessarily in pathological or traumatic situations). For example, in this conversation, "Yesterday I met a friend on the street and said, 'Hi, Brad, how are you?' And he said, 'Thank you, but my name is Fred!'" This is the percentage of false memories we observe, for example, at control subjects during the performance of a task on trials about false memories.

False memories are a consequence of how memories are built in the brain. Since the pioneering studies of Milner and her colleagues [33] on H.M., an amnesic patient who after the surgical resection of a large part of his medial temporal lobe presented many specific changes in his memory, the idea of memory as a single entity has been losing support. What was thought to be unique engrams of lived experiences has since then been broken down in a series of pieces that must be joined together to give rise to the experience of retrieving memories. Each one of these pieces is acquired with different codes and stored in different locations in the brain, depending on the different contexts in which they were obtained and in which they are recollected later. That is, the retrieval operation depends on the external and internal conditions at encoding and at retrieval. Memory cues remind details of the input occasion and are a necessary condition to the retrieval. Other external inputs like feelings, thoughts, and the motivational state are also very important for a true retrieval but sometimes may be not like the original situation.

In agreement with the conception that memory is composed of several systems, Brainerd and Reyna [34] proposed the fuzzy-trace theory (FTT). According to FTT, episodic memory consists of two independent and parallel subsystems called the literal system and essence. These two subsystems encode information in the form of different representations, constituting literal memory and memory of essence. While literal memory stores the specific and detailed traits of the episodes, the essence memory stores the nonspecific sense, e.g., the meaning, and the general patterns of the episodes. For the FTT, true memories are mostly due to the retrieval of literal memories. False memories, therefore, would be arising from the retrieval of memories of essence [35].

Traditionally, false memories have been investigated through various types of experimental procedures that enhance their occurrence, using materials such as slides, films, and sentences.

In the last decade, a widespread methodology is the list of associated words. This procedure, known by the acronym DRM, was developed by Roediger and McDermott [36] based on previous studies done by Deese many years before (1959). DRM consists of lists of words that are presented to be memorized (study phase) and later recognized (test phase). For this, standardized verbal stimuli (word lists) with neutral and emotional content (positive and negative) are adopted in a way to evaluate if the recognition was true or false, even if it is familiar or not. This method of organizing stimuli into thematically related sets was inspired by the previous research with words, which produced robust false recognition effects (see item 3).

It is thought that such false memories arise from the automatic activation of conceptually related words or "gist" information [37]. Thus, when reading the words in the study phase, people encode the target words through literal representations (specific and detailed characteristics, e.g., sound, spelling) and representations of essence (general characteristics and unspecific, e.g., the meaning). In the test phase, people recall or recognize the target words (true memory) by retrieving the literal and essence traces but recall or recognize the critical words (false memory) through retrieval only of essence traces. FTT has been widely used in interpreting results from research using the DRM procedure, for example, in studies that evaluated the effects of triazolam and scopolamine in the production of false memories for neutral words [38, 39].

In recognition tasks, in which the participants must distinguish items whose presentations are episodically remembered from those that seemed to be merely familiar that means they do not have a full memory. They recognize stimuli (words or images) previously presented (study phase) in a list that includes items that have not been presented before (recognition phase). Current models of recognition memory consider that recognition involves both familiarity and recollection. Familiarity seems to operate more quickly than the recollection, being defined as a quick decision of recognition. Some authors interpret the "remember" and "know" as responses that reflect different processes, of recollection and familiarity, respectively [40, 41].

The classification of stimuli in different emotional dimensions is also necessary, because some studies have shown that valence and the arousal influence the indexes of retrieval through different cognitive processes and neural mechanisms [42, 43]. It is assumed that valence and the arousal improve recollection, while the arousal increases familiarity [14]. On the other hand, true memories (events or thoughts) are often associated with retrieved experiences and feelings of familiarity, while false memories are characterized by feeling familiarity and no distinct state of consciousness [44]. During a recognition test, a decision-making process occurs whose participants give a "remember" answer when they recognize items that are accompanied by a conscious retrieval of their occurrence during an episodic memory study. On the other hand, they give a "know" answer to those items that do not evoke any detail, but which are recognized by other bases. The detailed instructions given to the participants for the "remember-know" trial can be obtained in previous studies [41, 45].

3. Neuropsychology as clinical tools to true and false memory: evaluation and rehabilitation

3.1. Evaluation

Some tests are classically used to evaluate false memory. One of them (cited above) is the *DRM*, a recognition test that associates words with neutral and emotional content. Each list contains 15 words (it may change depending on the study), and the words commonly chosen are those with the highest rates of false recognition. The word lists comprised some positive (e.g., music, fruit, sweet, and sleep), some neutral (e.g., chair, cold, pen, and high), and other negative contents (e.g., thief, trash, pain, and fear). The presentation order of the words is randomly generated and varied for each subject. The participants are instructed to encode all lists. The words of each list revolve around a theme in which it is strongly associated. These words were termed critical keywords [e.g., *smoke* (critical word), for which associated words that belong to a common theme are cigarette, puff, blaze, billows, pollution, ashes, cigar, chimney, fire, tobacco, stink, pipe, lungs, flames, and stain] that were the related lures. The critical word, smoke, that translates the thematic essence of the list and is semantically associated with all other words of the list is not presented in the memorization stage (study phase). The word *smoke* is remembered or recognized many times in the same proportion as words from the list studied.

The recognition task is carried out immediately (hours, days, etc.) after presentation of lists. It consists of 90 words, of which 45 of them are targets, 15 related lures, and 30 unrelated lures. The targets are the studied words in the original material taken from positions 1, 8, and 10 of the lists (hit rates); the related lures are words not presented in the original material but represent the semantic essence of each of the lists (false alarm); and the unrelated lures are words not presented in the original material that have no semantic relationship with them (response bias measured by item intrusions). The subjects were asked to circle the words, presented in a sheet of paper that they thought to have seen before. If they circle a target, the measure is considered a "hit rate," and if they circle a related lure, it is considered a "false alarm."

Another task to evaluate visual false memory is the *DRM-IAPS*, developed according to the same criterion of DRM paradigm adapted for the construction of a set of associated images from the International Affective Picture System (IAPS) [46]. The IAPS in turn must be standardized according to each population studied since it may vary according to it. It evaluates the emotional memory, constituting an adequate task to evaluate false memories.

As the DRM task, the DRM-IAPS (**Figure 4**) consists of two phases: the study phase (encoding) and recognition phase (recognition). The study phase consisted of 20 blocks with 6 pictures

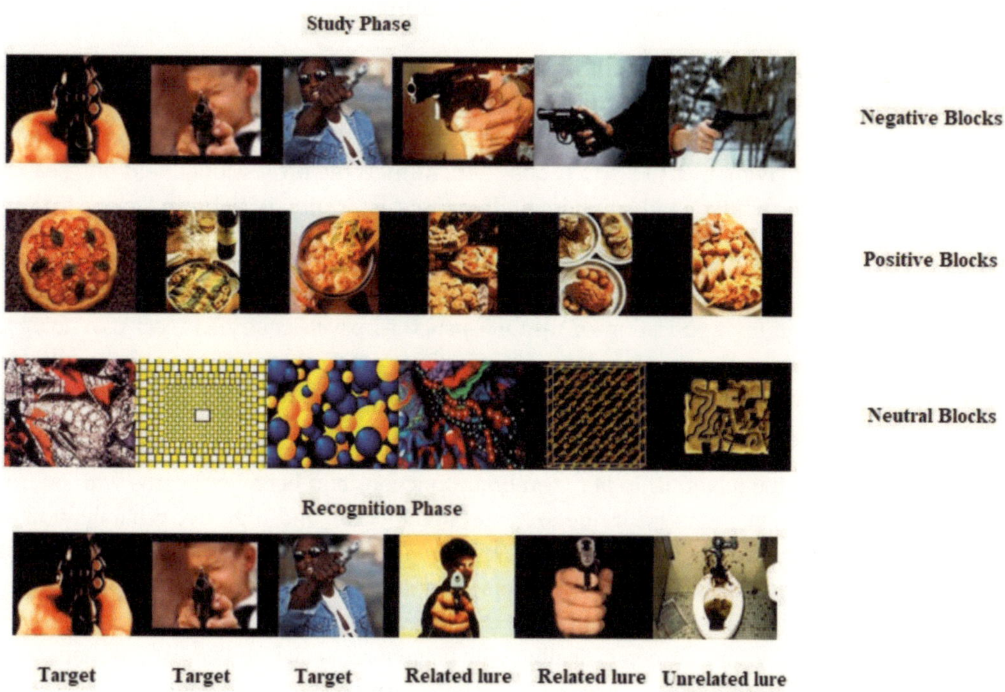

Figure 4. Example of DRM-IAPS task blocks (negative, positive, and neutral valences). Study and recognition phases.

that were elaborated, having a total of 120 photos (it may change according to the trial). The images are taken from the IAPS, which contains hundreds of color photographs capable of eliciting various emotional states. These images range from pleasant to unpleasant, arousal or relaxing, or neutral. The picture valence may be positive (e.g., food, sports, sex, etc.) or negative (e.g., guns, mutilated bodies, violence, and accidents). Each photograph, taken from the IAPS, showed a certain level of arousal and valence, whose average is calculated for each of the 20 blocks. These visual stimuli can induce various emotional states and represent many aspects of real life, sports, fashion, natural disasters, accidents, landscapes, pornography, violence, etc. and act as powerful generators of emotions easily presented in the experimental laboratory context, thus, allowing accurate control of their timing and exposure time.

So, usually most of the tasks aimed to study false memories consist of two phases: (1) the *encoding phase* (or study phase) and (2) *retrieval phase* (recognition or free recall phase test). During the recognition task, the subject may decide if they have seen the picture (stimulus) before or not. "Yes" responses to targets provided an index of true recognition, whereas "yes" responses to related lures provided an index of false recognition. During the recognition phase, it is also possible to evaluate the level of confidence of responses ("know/remember" answers). Physiological measures outcoming from emotional responses according to valence as well as arousal of the stimuli are commonly taken.

Other common tasks used on trials aimed to study false memories are as follows: emotional responses to pictures IAPS, personality trait of words, recognition of facial emotions, or films [46–50].

3.2. Neuropsychology and neuropsychological rehabilitation

The main role of neuropsychology is the evaluation of cognitive functions and their relation to behavior, which means to investigate the cerebral changes and their impact on the behavior of the individual. Neuropsychology is, in a broad sense (latus), the study of the relations between the brain and the behavior and, in a strict sense (strictum), is the professional field of research that investigates the cognitive and behavioral alterations associated with brain lesions [51].

Neuropsychology involves various types of knowledge such as neuroanatomy, neurophysiology, neurochemistry, and neuropharmacology, which contributes to the professional performance of the psychologist in the application of resources such as psychometry, clinical psychology, experimental psychology, psychopathology, and cognitive psychology. It is aimed to investigate cognitive functions such as memory, language, attention, executive function, perception, praxis, gnosis, mood, and personality disorders [52].

This investigation of the relationship between brain functions and behavior begins with neuropsychological evaluation, thenceforth due to neuropsychological and cognitive rehabilitation to be taken. Cognitive and neuropsychological rehabilitation are part of the field of psychology, first aimed to enable both patients and family members to minimize or overcome the cognitive deficits resulting from neurological disorders (acquired or congenital) and then the search for strategies for treatment of cognitive impairments, dealing with behavioral, social, and emotional changes in a way to improve quality of life of the patient [51]. There are many cognitive intervention technologies used as an aid to neuropsychological rehabilitation of the patient with different disorders such as temporal lobe epilepsy, schizophrenia, and stroke, among others. Varied from the simple the use of notes that help, for example, a patient with schizophrenia to remind their activities and commitments, until memory training, brain training, computerized exercises, and so on.

Just recently the researchers began to analyze false memories in pathological conditions (e.g., schizophrenia, post-traumatic stress disorder, and dementia) [53–56]. There are still many doubts to be elucidated in this fascinating area, and therefore the rehabilitation interventions are still to be defined in the next years.

4. Neuropharmacology on memory and false memories (dopaminergic modulation and other systems)

4.1. Dopaminergic modulation of true memories

The prefrontal cortex plays an essential role in the mediation of working memory, which has been observed in neuroimaging and neurophysiology studies, in monkeys and humans [57, 58]. Studies have demonstrated dopaminergic modulation of executive functions, working memory, and emotion [59, 60]. Studies with monkeys have shown that activation of dopamine D_1 receptors in the prefrontal cortex is necessary for the expression of working memory [57, 61]. Also, in humans, there is evidence of the predominant role of dopamine D_1 receptor with working memory [57, 62]. However, other studies with dopaminergic D_2 receptor antagonists and agonists have shown that they are also implicated in working memory in humans and monkeys [63–65]. According to Takahashi and colleagues, hippocampal D_2 receptors also influence frontal lobe functions, such as executive functions and verbal fluency [66]. Studies have particularly demonstrated the involvement of dopamine D_2 receptors in working memory, executive functions, working memory capacity, selective attention, and shifting [67–69]. Studies suggest that dopaminergic D_1 and D_2 receptors have complementary functions [70, 71].

Dopaminergic modulation of episodic memory was observed in humans [72]. Decreased binding to D_2 dopaminergic receptors in the hippocampus has been implicated in impairment of memory performance and learning impairments in Alzheimer's patients [73–75] and in experimental animals [76, 77]. There are many studies in humans and animals aimed to verify the involvement of dopamine in attentional mechanisms, executive functions, and working memory. Although the literature involving dopamine and emotion when referring to reward and addiction mechanisms is ample, few studies have evaluated the influence of dopaminergic receptors on emotional episodic memory.

Some neurological and psychiatric pathologies such as Parkinson's disease, schizophrenia, autism, attention deficit, Huntington's disease, and lesions of the frontal lobe present emotional process impairments. All these pathologies involve the dopaminergic system that suggests the participation of dopamine in emotion [78–83]. Moreover, emotional processes depend on different structures; many of them comprise the limbic system that has dopaminergic innervation. Many biochemicals, pharmacological, and neuroimaging studies reinforce the idea of dopaminergic contribution in emotion. A study with Parkinson's disease suggests that an abnormal state of the dopaminergic system compromises the normal operation of the amygdala) [21]. Some studies suggest the participation of dopaminergic D_2 receptors in emotional memory [84, 85].

The evaluation of the effect of specific drugs acting on several neurotransmitter systems on the functioning of memory for emotional stimuli is relevant, since healthy people process emotional episodes differently from episodes without emotional content. This often results in a higher probability of emotional events being retrieved than neutral ones [14, 86, 87]. The finding that emotions impact the performance of episodic memory has led some researchers to investigate the influence of emotions on the production of false memories. Although these researches present different results, perhaps stemming from a variety of methods employed, they all suggest that emotion interferes with the indices of false memories.

4.2. Dopaminergic and other neurotransmitter system modulation of false memories

Two studies using antipsychotics haloperidol and sulpiride, both dopamine D_2 receptor antagonists, set up to evaluate the dopaminergic modulation of false memories observed that the drugs increased false memory rates but had no effect on true memory [88, 89].

Other neurotransmitter system effects on the production of false memories were studied in trials with dextroamphetamines, Δ(9)-tetrahydrocannabinol (THC), and benzodiazepines (diazepam and lorazepam). The effect of caffeine and of alcohol on true and false memories was also investigated.

Ballard observed that dextroamphetamine (AMP) increases errors during memory retrieval [90]. The same author in another study found that AMP increases true, but not false, memory relative to placebo, but AMP increases false memory compared to THC [91]. In 1999, Blair and Curran observed that diazepam selectively impaired subjects' ability to recognize angry expressions but did not affect recognition of any other facial emotional expression [92]. A study demonstrated that diazepam and lorazepam impair conscious recollection associated with true, but not false, memories [93]. Caffeine appears to intensify the strength of connections among the list words and critical lures, thereby enhancing both true and false memories [94].

In 2012, another study observed more false-positive responses of ecstasy/polydrug users than nonusers [95]. Increased long-term frequency of ecstasy use was positively associated with memories when ingested before encoding. But differently it verified an increased false recognition when amphetamine was ingested before retrieval. On the contrary, alcohol appears to decrease semantic activation leading to a decline in false memories and decrease in rejection of false memories, commonly observed in placebo. The latter effect of alcohol may be due to its ability to impair monitoring processes established at encoding [96]. Milani and Curran compared the effect of low dose with high dose of alcohol on recollective experience of illusory memory [97]. They found high levels of false recall and recognition across both treatments and verified that a small dose of alcohol did not change too much measures of false memory but modifies the pattern of recollective experience in terms of remember and know responses. Specifically, it increased the level of remember responses for false recognitions (critical lures).

An autobiographical study reported that compared to placebo, lorazepam increased levels of conscious recollection, as assessed by "remember" responses, for both true and false memories and induced an overestimation of the personal significance and emotional intensity of past events [98].

Emotion facilitates true memory performance in comparison to neutral content events. However, in situations with negative emotional content, where the level of stress and cortisol released is high, the opposite must occur; that is, there is an impairment in the performance of processes such as perception and memory. This mechanism can be represented in a graph by one of the inverted "U" curves. These situations of high stress would be represented in the descending part of the curve, which means that the emotion has a facilitating effect on the encoding, but if the level of emotion is exaggerated, the effect is the contrary [99]. Possibly, at extreme stressful circumstances, with a high level of attention and arousal, an exaggerated processing of the relevant stimuli of the event (the central aspects) in detriment of the processing of peripheral (irrelevant) stimuli occurs. This unbalance during encoding could facilitate the formation of false memories through errors during the re-encoding of some memory traces.

Some possible mechanisms of dopaminergic modulation of false memories proposed by this chapter's authors would be (1) the dopamine effect on working memory/executive functions through corticostriatal as well as hippocampus-prefrontal D_2 dopaminergic modulation, (2) through D_2 dopaminergic modulation of the response of the amygdala to emotionally loaded stimuli, and (3) dopaminergic modulation of decision-making process (via striatum). Other possible failures in post-encoding through other neurotransmitters may also contribute to false memory formation. But the exact mechanisms as well as the role of other neurotransmitter systems on the production of false memories remain still to be clarified in the future.

5. Conclusions

The activation (agonism) or blockade (antagonism) of receptors may have different effects on emotional judgment of the stimulus and may stimulate or impair true or false memories depending on the drug and system studied. The study of false memories is a challenging area of neuroscience that is extraordinarily fascinating with many questions yet to be clarified in a way that in the future new methods and tools of neuropsychological rehabilitation can be proposed.

Conflict of interest

There is no conflict of interest.

Author details

Regina Vieira Guarnieri[1*], Orlando Francisco Amodeo Bueno[1] and Ivanda de Souza Silva Tudesco[1,2]

*Address all correspondence to: vguarnieri@uol.com.br

1 Department of Psychobiology, Universidade Federal de São Paulo, São Paulo, SP, Brazil

2 Psychology-Psychosomatics of Universidade Ibirapuera, São Paulo, SP, Brazil

References

[1] Squire LR, Kandel ER. Brain system from declarative memory. In: Scientific American Library, editor. Memory: From Mind to Molecules. New York; 1999. pp. 83-107

[2] Miyake A, Shah P, editors. Models of Working Memory: Mechanisms of Active Maintenance and Executive Control. New York: Cambridge University Press; 1999

[3] James W. The Principles of Psychology. Dover Publications; 1890 (1950, Vol. 1: ISBN: 0-486-20381-6, Vol. 2: ISBN 0-486-20382-4)

[4] Atkinson RC, Shiffrin RM. The control of short-term memory. Scientific American. 1971; **225**:82-90

[5] Cowan N. The magical number 4 in short-term memory: A reconsideration of mental storage capacity. Behavioral and Brain Sciences. 2000;**24**:87-185

[6] Baddeley AD, Hitch GJ. Working memory. In: Bower GA, editor. The Psychology of Learning and Motivation. New York: Academic Press; 1974. pp. 49-79

[7] Baddeley AD. Short-term and working memory. In: Tulving E, Craik FIM, editors. The Oxford Handbook of Memory. New York: Oxford University Press; 2000. pp. 77-92

[8] Baddeley AD, Della Sala S. Working memory and executive control. In: Roberts AC, Robbins TW, Weisenkrantz L, editors. The Prefrontal Cortex. Oxford: Oxford University Press; 1998. pp. 9-21

[9] Squire LR, Zola-Morgan S. The medial temporal lobe memory system. Science. 1991;**253**: 1380-1386

[10] Squire LR. Memory systems of the brain: A brief history and current perspective. Neurobiology of Learning and Memory. 2004;**82**:171-177

[11] Tulving E. Elements of Episodic Memory. New York: Oxford University Press; 1983

[12] Bradley MM, Lang PJ. Measuring emotion: The self-assessment manikin and semantic differential. Journal of Behavioral Therapy and Experimental Psychiatry. 1994;**25**(1):49-59

[13] Lang PJ. Behavioral treatment and bio-behavioral assessment: Computer applications. In: Sidowski JB, Johnson JH, Williams TA, editors. Technology in Mental Health Care Delivery Systems. Norwood, NJ: Ablexs; 1980. pp. 119-137

[14] Kensinger EA, Corkin S. Memory enhancement for emotional words: Are emotional words more vividly remembered than neutral words? Memory & Cognition. 2003;**31**(8): 1169-1180

[15] Burke A, Heuer F, Reisberg D. Remembering emotional events. Memory & Cognition. 1992;**20**:277-290

[16] Reisberg D, Heuer F. Memory for emotional events. In: Reiberg D, Hertel P, editors. Memory and Emotion. New York: Oxford University Press; 2004. pp. 3-41

[17] Hamann S. Cognitive and neural mechanisms of emotional memory. Trends in Cognitive Sciences. 2001;**5**:394-400

[18] Hamann SB, Cahill I, McGaugh JL, Squire IR. Intact enhancement of declarative memory for emotional material in amnesia. Learning & Memory. 2009;**4**:301-309

[19] Phelps EA. The human amygdala awareness: Interactions between emotion and cognition. In: Gazzanica MS, editor. The Cognitive Neuroscience III. Cambridge, MA: MIT press; 2004. pp. 1005-1016

[20] Hamann SB, Lee GP, Adolphs R. Impaired declarative emotional memory but intact emotional response following human bilateral amygdalobotomy. Society for Neuroscience. 1999;**25**:99 (abstract)

[21] Tessitore A, Hariri AR, Fera F, Smith WG, Chase TN, Hyde TM, et al. Dopamine modulates the response of the human amygdala: A study in Parkinson's disease. The Journal of Neuroscience. 2002;**22**(20):9099-9103

[22] Mcgaugh JL. The amygdala modulates the consolidation of memories of emotionally arousing experiences. Annual Review of Neuroscience. 2004;**27**:1-28

[23] Bechara A, Tranel D, Damasio H, Adolphs R, Rockland C, Damasio AR. Double dissociation of conditioning and declarative knowledge relative to the amygdala and hippocampus in humans. Science. 1995;**269**:1115-1118

[24] Pessoa I, Mckenna M, Gutierrez E, Ungerleider IG. Neural processing of emotional faces requires attention. Proceedings of the National Academy of Sciences of the United States of America. 2002;**99**:11458-11463

[25] Lane RD, Reiman EM, Axelrod B, Yun LS, Holmes A, Schwartz GE. Neural correlates of levels of emotional awareness: Evidence of an interaction between emotion and attention in the anterior cingulate cortex. Journal of Cognitive Neuroscience. 1998:525-535

[26] Bush G, Luu P, Posner MI. Cognitive and emotional influence of anterior cingulated cortex. Trends in Cognitive Sciences. 2000;**4**:215-222

[27] Rauch SI, Van der Kolk BA, Fisler RE, Alpert NM, et al. A symptom provocation study of posttraumatic disorder using positron emission tomography and script-driven imagery. Archives of General Psychiatry. 1996;**53**:380-390

[28] Damasio AR. The somatic markers hypothesis and the possible functions of the prefrontal cortex. Philosophical Transactions of the Royal Society of London. Series B, Biological Sciences. 1996;**351**:1413-1420

[29] Davidson RJ, Lewis DA, Alloy IB, Amaral DG, et al. Neural and behavioral substrates of mood and mood regulation. Society of Biological Psychiatry. 2002;**52**:478-502

[30] Lindsay DS. Contextualizing and clarifying criticisms of memory work in psychotherapy. Consciousness and Cognition. 1994;**3**:426-434

[31] Eisen MI, Quas JA, Goodman GS. In: Eisen MI, Quas JA, Goodman GS, editors. Memory and Suggestibility in the Forensic Interview. Mahwah (NJ): Lawrence Erlbaum; 2002

[32] Berntsen D. Tunnel memories for autobiographical events: Central details are remembered more frequently from shocking than from happy experiences. Memory & Cognition. 2002;**30**(7):1010-1020

[33] Scoville WB, Milner B. Loss of recent memory after bilateral hippocampal lesions. Journal of Neurology, Neurosurgery and Psychiatry. 1957;**20**:11-21

[34] Brainerd CJ, Reyna VF. Theorical explanation of false memories. In: Brainerd CJ, Reyna VF, editors. The Science of False Memory. Oxford: New York; 2005. pp. 59-96

[35] Brainerd CJ, Reyna VF. Fuzzy-trace and false memory. Current Direction in Psychological Science. 2002;**11**(5):164-168

[36] Roediger HI, Mcdermott KB. Creating false memories: Remembering words not presented on lists. Journal of Experimental Psychology: Learning, Memory, and Cognition. 1995;**21**(4):803-814

[37] Schacter DL, Slotnick SD. The cognitive neuroscience of memory distortion. Neuron. 2004;**44**:149-160

[38] Mintzer MZ, Griffiths RR. False recognition in triazolam-induced amnesia. Journal of Memory and Language. 2001;**44**:475-492

[39] Mintzer MZ, Griffiths RR. Acute dose-effects of scopolamine on false recognition. Psychopharmacology. 2001;**153**:425-433

[40] Conway MA, Dewhurst SA. Remembering, familiarity and source monitoring. Quarterly Journal of Experimental Psychology. 1995;**48A**:125-114

[41] Gardiner JM. Functional aspects of recollective experience. Memory & Cognition. 1988; **16**:309-313

[42] Kensinger EA. Remembering emotional experiences: The contribution of valence and arousal. Reviews in the Neurosciences. 2004;**15**:241-251

[43] Kensinger EA, Corkin S. Two routes of emotional memory: Distinct neural processes for valence and arousal. Proceedings of the National Academy of Sciences of the United States of America. 2004;**101**(9):3310-3315

[44] Conway MA, Collins AF, Gathercole ES, Anderson SJ. Recollections of true and false memories. Journal of Experimental Psychology, General. 1996;**125**(1):69-95

[45] Rajaram S. Perceptual effects on remembering: Recollective processes in picture recognition memory. Journal of Experimental Psychology: Learning, Memory, and Cognition. 1996;**22**:365-377

[46] Lang PJ, Bradley MM, Cuthbert BN. International affective picture system (IAPS): Inst ruction manual and affective ratings. Technical Report A-4. The Center for Research in Psychophysiology, University of Florida. 1997

[47] Anderson NH. Likableness ratings of 555 personality-trait words. Journal of Personality and Social Psychology. 1968;**9**:272-279

[48] Ekman P, Friesen WV. Pictures of Facial Affect [Slides]. Palo Alto, CA: Consulting Psychologists Press; 1976

[49] Harmer CJ, Shelley NC, Cowen PJ, et al. Increased positive versus negative affective perception and memory in healthy volunteers following selective serotonin and norepinephrine reuptake inhibition. American Journal of Psychiatry. 2004;**161**:1256-1263

[50] Quevedo J, Sant'Anna MK, Madruga M, Lovato I, de-Paris F, Kapczinski F, et al. Differential effects of emotional arousal in short and long-term memory in healthy adults. Neurobiology of Learning and Memory. 2003;**79**(2):132-135

[51] Hamdan AC, Pereira APA, Riechi TIJS. Avaliação e reabilitação neuropsicológica: desenvolvimento histórico e perspectivas atuais. Interação em Psicologia. 2011;**15**:47-58

[52] Lezak MD, Howieson DB, Loring DW. Neuropsychological Assessment. 4th ed. New York: Oxford University Press; 2004

[53] Fairfield B, Altamura M, Padalino FA, Balzotti A, Di Domenico A, Nicola Mammarella N. False memories for affective information in schizophrenia. Frontiers in Psychiatry. 2016; **7**(191):1-9. DOI: 10.3389/fpsyt.2016.00191

[54] Moradi AR, Heydari AH, Abdollahi MH, Rahimi-Movaghar V, Dalgleish T, Jobson L. Visual false memories in posttraumatic stress disorder. Journal of Abnormal Psychology. 2015;**124**(4):905-917. DOI: 10.1037/abn0000109

[55] Hayes JP, LaBar KS, Nasser J, Dolcos F. Reduced hippocampal and amygdala activity predicts memory distortions for trauma reminders in combat-related PTSD. Journal of Psychiatry Research. 2011;**45**(5):660-669. DOI: 10.1016/j.jpsychires.2010.10.007

[56] Phillipps C, Kemp J, Jacob C, Veronneau A, et al. Comparative study of false memory in dementia with Lewy bodies and Alzheimer's disease. Geriatrie et Psychologie Neuropsychiatrie du Vieillissement. 2016;**14**(3):332-340. DOI: 10.1684/pnv.2016.0620

[57] Sawaguchi T, Goldman-Rakik PS. D1 dopamine receptors in prefrontal cortex: Involvement in working memory. Science. 1991;**251**:947-950

[58] Arnsten AFT, Cai JX, Murphy Bl, Goldman-Rakic PS. Dopamine D1 receptor mechanisms in the cognitive performance of young adult aged monkeys. Psychopharmacology. 1994;**11**:143-151

[59] Floresco SB, Magyar O. Mesocortical dopamine modulation of executive functions: Beyond working memory. Psychopharmacology. 2006;**188**:567-555

[60] Nieoullon A, Coquerel A. Dopamine: A key regulator to adapt action, emotion, motivation and cognition. Current Opinion in Neurology. 2009;**16**(Suppl 2):S3-S9

[61] Wang K, Hoosain R, Yang RM, et al. Impairment of recognition of disgust in Chinese with Huntington's or Wilson's disease. Neuropsychologia. 2003;**41**:527-537

[62] Müller U, Yves von Cramon D, Pollmann S. D1- versus D2-receptor modulation of visuospatial working memory in humans. The Journal of Neuroscience. 1998;**18**(7):2720-2728

[63] Arnsten AFT, Cai JX, Steere JC, Goldman-Rakik PS. Dopamine D2 receptors mechanisms contribute to age-related cognitive decline: The effects of quinpirole on memory and motor performance in monkeys. Journal of Neuroscience. 1995;**15**:3429-3439

[64] Luciana M, Depue RA, Arbisi P, Leon A. Facilitation of working memory in humans by a D2 dopamine receptor agonist. Journal of Cognitive Neuroscience. 1992;**4**:58-67

[65] Mehta MA, Hinton EC, Montgomery AJ, Bantick RA, Grasby PM. Sulpiride and mnemonic function: Effects of a dopamine D_2 receptor antagonist on working memory, emotional

memory and long-term memory in healthy volunteers. Journal of Psychopharmacology. 2005;**19**:29-38

[66] Takahashi H, Kato M, Hayashi M, Okubo Y, Takano A, Ito H, et al. Memory and frontal lobe functions; possible relations with dopamine D2 receptors in the hippocampus. NeuroImage. 2007;**34**:1643-1649

[67] Mehta MA, Manes FF, Magnolfi G, Sahakian BJ, Robbins TW. Impaired set-shifting and dissociable effects on tests of spatial working memory following the dopamine D2 receptor antagonist sulpiride in human volunteers. Psychopharmacology. 2004;**176**:331-334

[68] Ward R, Duncan J, Shapiro K. The slow time-course of visual attention. Cognitive Psychology. 1996;**30**:79-109

[69] Kimberg DY, D'Esposito M, Farah MJ. Effects of bromocriptine depends on working memory capacity. Neuroreport. 1997;**8**(16):3581-3585

[70] Barone P, Palma V, DeBartolomeis A, Tedeschi E, Muscettola G, Campanella G. Dopamine D1 and D2 receptors mediate opposite functions in seizures induced by lithium-pilocarpine. European Journal of Pharmacolology. 1991;**195**:157-162

[71] Bo P, Soragna D, Marchioni E, Candeloro E, Albergati A, Savoldi F. Role of dopamine D-1 and D-2 antagonists in a model of focal epilepsy induced by electrical stimulation of hippocampus and amygdala in the rabbit. Progress in Neuropsychopharmacology and Biological Psychiatry. 1995;**19**:917-930

[72] Schott H, Seidenbercher C, Fenker DB, Lauer CJ, Bunzeck N, Bernstein H-G, et al. The dopaminergic midbrain participates in human episodic memory formation: Evidence from genetic imaging. Journal of Neuroscience. 2006;**26**:1407-1417

[73] Joyce JN, Kaeger C, Ryoo H, Goldsmith S. Dopamine D2 receptors in the hippocampus and amygdala in Alzheimer's disease. Neuroscience Letters. 1993;**154**:171-174

[74] Kemppainen N, Laine M, Laakso MP, Kaasinen V, Nagren K, Vahlberg T, et al. Hippocampal dopamine D2 receptors correlate with memory functions in Alzheimer's disease. European Journal of Neuroscience. 2003;**18**:149-154

[75] Reeves S, Mehta M, Howard R, Grasby P, Brown R. The dopaminergic basis of cognitive and motor performance in Alzheimer's disease. Neurobiology of Disease. 2010;**37**:477-482

[76] Fujishiro H, Umegaki H, Suzuki Y, Oohara-Kurotani S, Yamaguchi Y, Iguchi A. Dopamine D2 receptor plays a role in memory function: Implications of dopamine-acetylcholine interaction in the ventral hippocampus. Psychopharmacology. 2005;**182**:253-261

[77] Umegaki H, Munoz J, Meyer RC, Spangler EL, Yoshimura J, Ikari H, et al. Involvement of dopamine D2 receptors in complex maze learning and acetylcholine release in ventral hippocampus of rats. Neuroscience. 2001;**103**:27-33

[78] Dujardin K, Blairy S, Defrebve L, et al. Subthalamic nucleus stimulation induces deficits in decoding emotional facial expressions in Parkinson's disease. Journal of Neurological Neurosurgery Psychiatry. 2004;**75**:202-208

[79] Bryson G, Bell M, Lysaker P. Affect recognition in schizophrenia: A function of global impairment or a specific cognitive deficit. Psychiatry Research. 1997;**71**:105-113

[80] Volkmar FR. Pharmacological intervention in autism: Theoretical and practical issues. Journal of Clinical Child Psychology. 2001;**30**:80-87

[81] Rapport LJ, Friedman SR, Tzelepis A, et al. Experienced emotion and affect recognition in adult attention-deficit hyperactivity disorder. Neuropsychology. 2002;**16**:102-110

[82] Backman L, Farde L. Dopamine and cognitive functioning: Brain imaging findings in Huntington's disease and normal aging. Scandinavian Journal of Psychology. 2001;**42**: 2870-2296

[83] Lee MJ, Swann AC, Dafny N. Methylphenidate sensitization is prevented by prefrontal cortex lesion. Brain Research Bulletin. 2008;**76**:131-140

[84] McDowell S, Whyte J, D'Esposito M. Differential effect of a dopaminergic agonist on prefrontal function in traumatic brain injury patients. Brain. 1998;**121**:1155-1164

[85] Powell JH, al-Adawi S, Morgan J, et al. Motivational deficits after brain injury: Effects of bromocriptine in 11 patients. Journal of Neurology, Neurosurgery, and Psychiatry. 1996; **60**:416-421

[86] LaBar KS, Phelphs EA. Arousal-mediated memory consolidation: Role of the medial temporal lobe in humans. Psychological Science. 1998;**9**(6):490-493

[87] Ochsner KN. Are affective events richly recollected or simply familiar? The experience and process of recognizing feelings past. Journal of Experimental Psychology: General. 2000; **129**(2):242-261

[88] Guarnieri RV, Buratto LG, Gomes CFA, Ribeiro RL, deSousa AAL, Stein LM, et al. Haloperidol increases false recognition memory of thematically related pictures in healthy volunteers. Human Psychopharmacology: Clinical and Experimental. 2016;**32**:e2563. DOI: 10.1002/hup.2563

[89] Guarnieri RV, Ribeiro RL, De Souza AA, Galduróz JF, Covolan L, Bueno OFA. Effects of sulpiride on true and false memories of thematically related pictures and associated words in healthy volunteers. Frontiers in Psychiatry. 2016;**7**:28. DOI: 10.3389/fpsyt.2016.00028

[90] Ballard M, Gallo D, de Wit H. Amphetamine increases errors during episodic memory retrieval. Journal of Clinical Psychopharmacology. 2014;**34**:85-92. DOI: 10.1097/ JCP.000 0000000000039

[91] Ballard M, Gallo D, de Wit H. Psychoactive drugs and false memory: Comparison of dextroamphetamine and delta-9-tetrahydrocannabinol on false recognition. Psychopharmacology. 2012;**219**:15-24. DOI: 10.1007/s00213-011-2374-5

[92] Blair RJR, Curran HV. Selective impairment in the recognition of anger induced by diazepam. Psychopharmacology. 1999;**147**:335-338

[93] Huron C, Servais C, Danion JM. Lorazepam and diazepam impair true, but not false, recognition in healthy volunteers. Psychopharmacology. 2001;**155**:204-209. DOI: 10.1007/s00 2130100683

[94] Capek S, Guenther RK. Caffeine's effects on true and false memory. Psychological Reports. 2009;**104**:787-795. DOI: 10.2466/PR0.104.3.787-795

[95] Gallagher DT, Fisk JE, Montgomery C, Judge J, Sarita J, Robinson SJ, et al. Effects of ecstasy/polydrug use on memory for associative information. Psychopharmacology. 2012;**222**:579-559. DOI: 10.1007/s00213-012-2652-x

[96] Garfinkel SN, Dienes Z, Duka T. The effect of alcohol and repetition at encoding on implicit and explicit false memories. Psychopharmacology. 2006;**188**(4):498-508. ISSN 0033-3158

[97] Milani R,·Curran HV. Effects of a low dose of alcohol on recollective experience of illusory memory. Psychopharmacology. 2000;**147**:397-402

[98] Pernot-Marino E, Danion JM, Hedelin G. Relations between emotion and conscious recollection of true and false autobiographical memories: An investigation using lorazepam as a pharmacological tool. Psychopharmacology. 2004;**175**(1):60-67

[99] Lupien SJ, Fiocco A, Wan N, Maheu F, Lord C, Schramek T, et al. Stress hormones and human memory function across the lifespan. Psychoneuroendocrinology. 2005;**30**:225-242